Mother & Baby

BABY MILESTONES

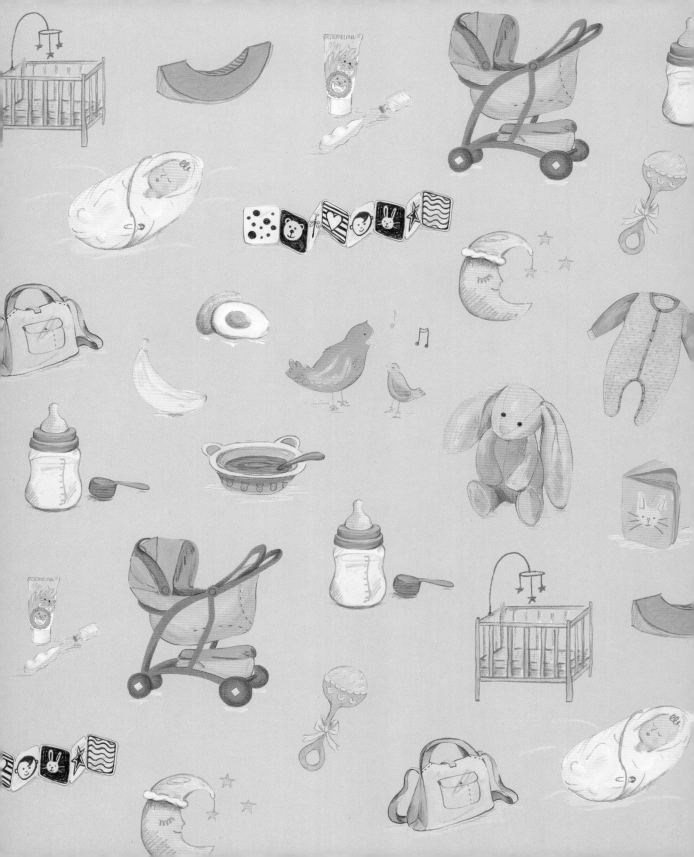

Mother & Baby

BABY MILESTONES

CONTRIBUTING EDITOR LARA PALAMOUDIAN

hamlyn

CONTENTS

LOOK OUT FOR THE TIMELINES...

to guide you through your child's exciting first year

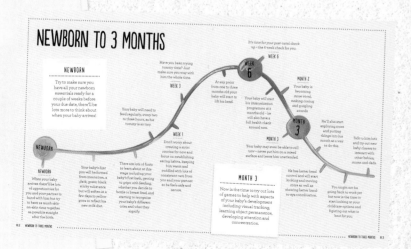

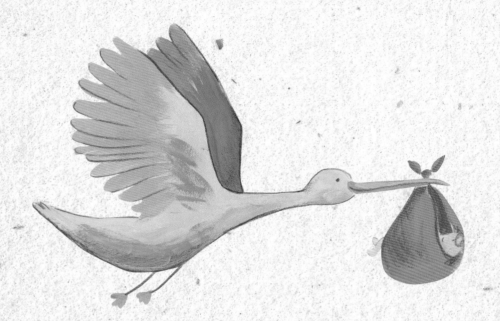

FOREWORD

Deciding to have a baby is one of the biggest decisions anyone will make and is life-changing in every way imaginable.

From the time you start trying to conceive until the precious moment you hold your little bundle of joy for the first time, you will be bombarded with a staggering amount of advice, whether it is from your mom, your best friend or the internet.

So while the journey to motherhood is an exciting experience, it is no surprise that it can also feel confusing and overwhelming as you try to work out the best choices for *you*.

At *Mother&Baby*, we have spent 60 years navigating women through pregnancy and early motherhood so our expertise is second to none. This is why we decided to put together these friendly, easy-to-read books. *Baby Milestones* covers everything you need to know about your baby's crucial first year and we are confident you will find it an invaluable guide throughout your incredible journey.

Enjoy!

The Mother&Baby team

INTRODUCTION

You've finally had your beautiful baby! No matter how long your pregnancy may have felt at the time, those nine months may feel like a distant memory now your little one is here. Soon he'll be hitting lots of important milestones—from sleeping through the night, teething, and weaning to crawling and walking.

Of course, all babies change and grow at different rates but we'll give you tips on what to look out for and how to help boost his development—both physically as well as through play and communication—during his first year. Read all about his first few hours as a newborn and the amazing things his body can do already, how you can help him learn more, the basics of caring for your little one, and read expert tips on managing his sleep and feeding routine (whether you're breast or bottle feeding).

As he develops, discover how he will change and how to help him learn about the world. We'll also be taking you through some practical information on keeping him healthy and happy.

As he becomes more mobile we'll give you tips on keeping him safe in your home and out and about. Of course, with age come changes in behavior and we'll help you manage those too—from trying to decipher his cries to how to cope with a full-on toddler tantrum in the supermarket (it happens!).

However, while it's essential to make sure your newborn is healthy and happy, it's also easy to forget about yourself in the midst of your new life as a mommy. But a confident, relaxed, happy mom makes for a happy baby—and you matter too. Which is why we're not only going to talk through those all-important developmental stages your baby is going through—we'll be carving out a little time to think about your needs as well in the Mama Zone.

Our practical and insightful expert advice will help you look after your mind and body now you're a mom—so while your real world support network will be there for you, we'll also be on hand to help with your emotions and your health in this first year. We'll help with bonding tips for both you and your partner, advice on making mommy friends, and support when it comes to those "Am I a good mom?" worries. We've got tips on staying healthy and feeling more energized (when you've had zero sleep) as well as getting your sex life on track. We've also got it covered when it comes to the practical stuff like working out when is the right time to go back to work (if and when you choose to) and finding the right childcare for your little one.

Please remember however, the advice and timelines in this book are simply guidelines and ideas, and not a substitute for medical advice—your baby is an individual, so talk to your pediatrician if you have any questions or worries about his development or health.

So, read on to find out more about your incredible baby, and your new life being a mom. Whatever your personal parenting style, we're here to help. Just remember, there's no such thing as the perfect parent—so don't be too hard on yourself at this new stage in your life. Giving your baby lots of love and being the best mom you can? Sounds good to us...

Lara Palamoudian
Contributing editor

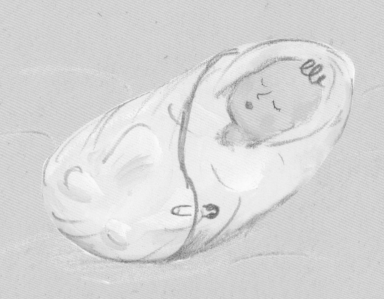

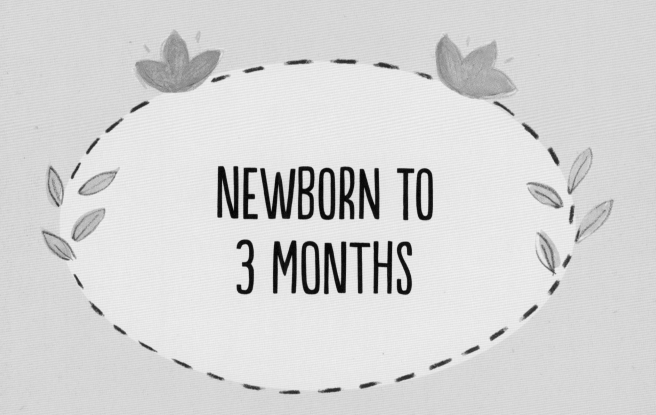

NEWBORN TO
3 MONTHS

YOUR FIRST HOURS TOGETHER

NEWBORN ESSENTIALS

FEEDING, WASHING, AND SLEEPING

CHAPTER ONE
A NEWBORN BABY

The arrival of your baby is the start of an amazing new way of life. The first 24 hours in particular will test you and your partner as you practise caring for your newborn, adjust to having her in your life and recover from giving birth.

A NEW FAMILY LIFE

At first there's the joy and excitement of having your baby, which may be tinged with worry at the responsibility. Your hormones will be fluctuating to accommodate the new challenge of looking after your baby, so you might feel tired and weepy one moment, then full of beans and positivity the next. This is normal in the early days. So what else can you expect on that first day?

YOUR FIRST HOURS TOGETHER

When your baby is first born, she will be given a quick wipe down to remove any amniotic fluid. The nurse will try not to remove too much of the vernix—the waxy substance that covers your baby—as it protects her skin in the first days.

Your baby will usually be placed straight onto your chest for skin-to-skin contact and maybe her first feed. She may spend around 20 minutes looking about or she may equally well fall asleep or start "rooting" for your breast.

Some babies latch on immediately, but many need help to get into position, and your nurse will advise. If you decide to bottle feed your baby, the hospital will supply you with bottles and formula—often, single-serve, ready-to-use containers—plus feeding advice. Always ask for help if you need it. After your baby has had skin-to-skin contact and a feed, your nurse will put her in a diaper.

The first sleep
Being born is exhausting for everyone, including your newborn, so don't be surprised if she falls asleep soon afterwards. This may sound like a good time for you to sleep too but, with all the hormones and adrenaline pumping around your body, it might not come easily. You should just try to rest and take it all in. Some pain-relief drugs you might have been given could make your baby drowsy too. However, even if she's sleepy, you may be advised to wake her for a feed every few hours (ask your nurse).

The first poo
At some point in the first 24 hours, your baby will have her first poo. Your nurse can show you how to change a diaper. Most hospitals will provide diapers, but pack some in your bag just in case. If you're not sure when to change your newborn, have a peek down the back of her diaper. Your baby's first bowel movements are a dark, green-black color and very sticky. This is called meconium. It is hard to clean off your baby's bottom, but after a few days her poo will change to a softer yellow to reflect her milk diet and it's much easier to clean off.

The first feeds
Your baby's tummy is small so she can't take much food and will need to feed approximately every three hours. The AAP states that breastfeeding is the healthiest way to feed your baby. Giving your baby breast milk exclusively is recommended for around the first six months. After that, giving breast milk alongside other food will help her continue to grow and develop healthily. Breast milk is the only natural food designed for your baby and protects her from infections and diseases. Breastfed babies have less chance of diarrhea and vomiting, fewer chest and ear infections, less chance of being constipated or developing eczema, and less likelihood of becoming obese (and developing obesity-related illnesses later in life). Any amount of breastfeeding has a positive effect and breast milk adapts as your baby grows to meet her needs. You'll be encouraged to breastfeed, however not all moms can or wish to. It can be a sensitive, emotional and personal decision so ditch the guilt, and do what is right for you and your baby.

GOING HOME WITH YOUR BABY

If your delivery is uncomplicated, your stay in hospital is likely to be short (many moms are discharged after two days) and you'll be ready for the drive home. Before you're discharged a pediatrician will check your baby over and the nurses should make sure you understand how to feed her. By law, you can't go home without a car seat and you'll have to show the hospital you have one (avoid a carpark grapple with the seat by fitting it beforehand). The car seat should click into the car seat base that you leave in the car, which you can attach to the car's LATCH system (fit in most cars manufactured since 2002). Check the latest guidelines and laws about baby seats, and ask which type of seat you need in advance—a reputable baby store will be able to help.

The first night
Your first night at home is both exciting and overwhelming. But remember, she'll sleep a lot at first, probably 15 hours a day, and she'll wake for feeds every two or three hours. Dress her and keep an eye on her temperature; you can check her temperature by feeling her stomach or the back of her neck. A newborn's circulation is slow, so her hands and feet may feel quite cool, but that doesn't mean she's cold. Keep a crib or Moses basket next to your bed so you can feed her easily. Place her in a special baby sleep sack to keep her warm. Never cover your baby with a blanket to provide warmth. (see guidelines for safe sleeping, page 24).

Getting some morning air
When you need some fresh air, and if you feel like venturing out for your first ever stroll with your baby, pack your diaper bag, burp cloths, and milk if you are bottle feeding, and pick a location close to home. Keep it easy and simple: going somewhere that doesn't involve transport will limit any stress and you can focus on getting some fresh air, stretching your legs and relaxing—your local park or café are good options. It's completely normal to feel anxious about introducing your baby to the big wide world, so consider taking your partner, mom or a friend to help you stay relaxed—and to be an extra pair of hands if you need one. See more about going out with your baby on page 43.

BONDING WITH YOUR BABY

You may think your little bundle just sleeps and feeds, but from day one she's soaking up information. She's already aware that her new surroundings—the outside world—are different from the womb, and she'll crave the environment

REAL LIFE

"I didn't feel an instant bond"

"I had a drawn out birth with Bobby and the doctors used forceps to ease him out, leaving me tired and bruised. Although I was so happy to finally meet him and loved him completely, I didn't feel an instant bond. Instead, our connection grew stronger steadily over hours, days, and weeks."

ABBIE, MOM TO BOBBY, TWO

she's enjoyed for the last nine months. She'll want to feel warm and safe so she'll probably just want to feed and be held a lot to start with.

Right from the beginning babies listen, watch and start to recognize people and objects (and from around the six-week mark, you may get that magical first smile, see page 45). Your baby can see for a distance of 10 to 12 inches but she can't see much further. She can make eye contact with you when she's feeding or with the person who's holding her. Her eyesight takes around six months to establish, so she'll be fascinated by very simple and contrasting patterns at this stage. Researchers at Stanford University have discovered that babies can make out a face at just an hour old—a newborn learns to recognize faces long before other objects. It's thought this is an instinct that helps with bonding. So keep your bond strong with lots of eye contact and close face-to-face time.

Postpartum depression can develop at any time during the first year after birth. If you are feeling low, talk to your family doctor, and be aware of the symptoms of postpartum depression—read more about it on page 54 and find more information at www.nimh.nih.gov/health/publications/postpartum-depression-facts.

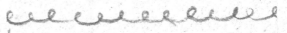

EXPERT TIP

MANAGING VISITORS

Your cellphone's probably been ringing constantly since your baby was born, but whether you want visitors is up to you. Try to make a plan in advance. For example, you may want to keep the first few days for yourself, and perhaps grandparents, and then have one visitor at a time after that. This gives you time to re-energize a little.

PENNY LAZELL
Healthcare professional

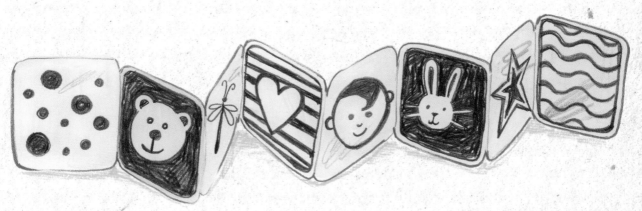

ESSENTIALS FOR YOUR NEWBORN

Here's a list of everything your baby needs in your first days together.

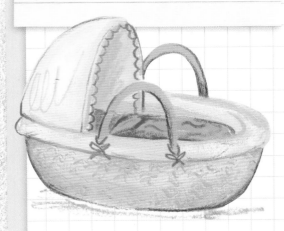

○ Food

While breastfeeding just requires boobs and a bra, if you're bottle-feeding you'll need at least three bottles (with newborn-sized nipples), a brush for washing the bottles, and the milk powder if you are feeding formula.

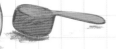

○ Clothes

A baby's capsule wardrobe should include enough T-shirts with snap fasteners and footsie pajamas. You'll need hats and a padded one-piece for going outside. Scratch mittens and socks are also useful.

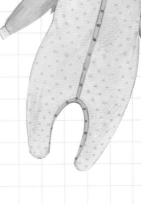

○ Somewhere to sleep

Your newborn can sleep in a crib, but she might find a bassinet cosier. Use a crib that meets current Consumer Product Safety Commission standards. Follow safe sleep guidelines set out on page 24 to minimize the risk of Sudden Infant Death Syndrome (SIDS).

○ Bedding

Use fitted sheets and never place flat sheets, blankets or pillows with your baby.

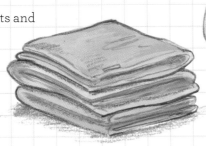

○ Bibs or burp cloths

You'll need at least six to soak up dribbles and post-feed spit-ups.

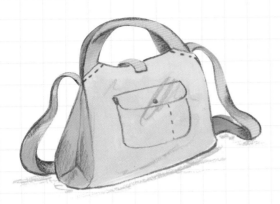

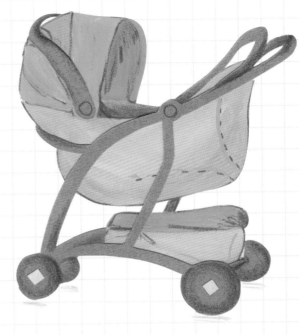

○ **Diaper bag**
The easiest way to keep your baby's kit together is to put everything in a diaper bag. Ideally choose one with a waterproof lining and lots of pockets. Alternatively, a large tote bag will do the job.

○ **Change mat, diapers, and cotton or babywipes**
Go for a newborn diaper size and you'll need lots of baby wipes and barrier cream.

○ **Car seat**
This is a legal requirement when you're bringing your baby home from hospital. Make sure you have worked out how to fix it in place before your baby is born.

○ **Baby pram or stroller**
You'll need to put your baby in a pram suitable for newborns. This means that the seat must recline to a reasonable degree, because newborn neck muscles aren't developed enough to allow for sitting (so jogging strollers are out for at least six months). Most baby strollers and traveling systems let you snap the baby's car seat securely onto the stroller, which makes it easy to transfer your baby without waking her from a nap. Don't let her sleep in her car seat regularly for long periods of time.

SO, HOW DO I LOOK AFTER A BABY?

Looking after a new baby can feel overwhelming as there's so much you have never done before. Like any new challenge, though, it is easier if you've brushed up on the skills you need beforehand. These days moms can be sent home from hospital very quickly after the birth, so it can feel as if you're thrown in at the deep end. You will go to visit your baby's new pediatrician in the first few days, but we've laid out the basic skills to get you through.

Dressing your new baby

It can be difficult to dress a newborn, but it gets easier. Sleeves seem to be the trickiest part. You can roll them up so you can just pass your baby's hand through the armhole, then pull the sleeve down. Practise on a teddy or doll to get the hang of it. Also, look out for clothes with large openings and poppers rather than buttons, which make dressing easier. Buy vests with special "envelope" necks so they can be removed top or bottom. Make sure your baby's babygros have lots of room around the feet so that her toes aren't constricted.

Dress your baby in light layers so you can keep her at a comfortable temperature; don't let her become too hot. To check, feel her tummy, chest or the back of her neck. Don't worry if her hands and feet are cool as that's perfectly normal.

HOW TO WASH YOUR BABY

Your baby's skin is delicate and it doesn't really get dirty so stick to plain water to clean her for the first few weeks, after which you can buy gentle baby toiletries. You don't need to give your baby a bath every day. It's enough to give her a sponge bath every day with warm water and a washcloth or cotton balls (see page 30).

HOW TO PICK UP YOUR BABY

The key to handling your newborn is ensuring her head is supported at all times. To lift your baby, place the palm of your hand under your baby's shoulders and support her head with your fingers, then shuffle your other hand underneath her body and bring her into the crook of your arm. She could wriggle so only lift her up when you're sure.

HOW TO CHANGE A DIAPER

Change your baby's diaper after every feed, or if it's soiled—this can be around 12 times in 24 hours when she's a newborn.

○ **Have everything you need within reach**
You'll need a clean diaper, baby wipes, plus a change of clothes just in case. A quarter of babies get diaper rash, so keep a barrier cream handy, too.

○ **Keep an eye on your baby at all times**
While newborns don't roll, they can make sudden movements, so for the first few weeks, change her on the floor or your bed (well away from the edge so she can't fall off).

○ **Lay your baby on the mat**
Undress her bottom half then undo the dirty diaper and, lifting the front, fold it down under your baby's bottom.

○ **Remove the diaper and clean her bottom**
Use a baby wipe, making sure to use a fresh one for every wipe. Wipe from front to back. If you have a boy, clean the folds around the scrotum, but don't pull the foreskin back. Some babies, especially boys, pee when they're exposed to the air, so be prepared to cover the stream. With girls, clean front to back as well so you don't introduce bacteria into the vaginal area. Clean around the labia, but never inside. Clean around the umbilical stump during diaper changes only if it has gotten soiled. Rubbing alcohol is good.

○ **Dry your baby**
Pat the skin dry with a burp cloth and smooth on a thin layer of a diaper cream that contains zinc oxide, if you can see the beginnings of a rash. Lift her legs up and place the fresh diaper underneath her bottom with the tabs at the back, level with her waist. With a boy, make sure the penis is pointing down (at six o'clock position) so he doesn't pee out of the diaper.

○ **Fix the diaper**
Bring the front part of the diaper forward and up to your baby's tummy (be careful of her umbilical stump, which will now be in the process of healing and drying up) and stick down the tabs. If your baby still has her umbilical cord attached, fold the top of the diaper down so it doesn't rub the stump. Check the diaper grips your baby's legs without rubbing and you're now ready to dress your baby.

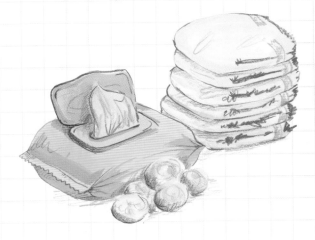

FEEDING YOUR BABY

Whether you choose to breastfeed your baby or bottle feed, or a combination of both, you'll spend a lot of time feeding so it's important to make the experience as relaxing and beneficial as possible for both of you.

HOW TO BURP YOUR BABY

After every feed, you need to spend some time freeing any air that your baby has gulped down with her milk or she could get tummy ache. Sit her upright on your lap, support her head and neck, and gently rub her back. Ask your pediatrician to show the safe way to get her in position if you're not sure. You could also try holding her against your shoulder gently rubbing her back. Listen out for burps—usually there's more than one. Change position regularly to help bring up the air. If you haven't heard a burp after ten minutes it's fine to stop.

HOW TO MAKE BREASTFEEDING EASIER

Breastfeeding can be an incredible bonding experience, and provides all the nutrition your baby needs (plus, it's free). Here are some tips:

❍ **Have skin-to-skin contact**
Make sure your doctor knows you want to breastfeed so she can help you have lots of skin-to-skin contact after birth. Studies suggest that if a baby is kept skin-to-skin with mom for an hour after birth she is likely to adjust to her new world more quickly and latch on well for feeding.

❍ **Ask for help**
See if a nurse or lactation consultant can be with you during your first few attempts at feeding; she can see if your baby is "latched on" properly. Bring your baby to your breast. Support her with your hand behind her shoulder blades and on the back of her neck, but don't hold the back of her head. Bring your baby towards your breast, aiming the nipple towards her nose (she will open her mouth when she senses your nipple on her lips). This will help her to take your areola into her mouth, and will position you inside her mouth correctly. Her cheeks should look full when she's feeding. If your baby cries or feeding

continues to hurt after the first few sucks she may not be latched on properly. At this point, get advice from your nurse; you may need to take your baby off the nipple (put your finger into one side of her mouth to break the suction) and start again. Offer the first breast, then if your baby relaxes and the nipple slips from her mouth, but she is still alert, offer the second—she may not want it, which is fine, but you're teaching her to take in what she needs.

Be aware of your let-down reflex

This happens when your muscles contract to release milk through your nipple and it can feel tingly. If your let-down is very fast, your baby may choke and splutter on your milk. If you're concerned that your baby is struggling with the rate of your milk flow, speak to your baby's pediatrician.

Look out for engorgement

As your breasts switch from making the first milk, colostrum, to mature milk (when your milk "comes in"), they can become swollen and solid, or engorged, which can be quite painful. Engorgement can be helped by a warm flannel or expressing, but the best solution is feeding, as missing feeds can trigger the condition, or expressing milk to relieve the pressure. If left, engorgement can turn into mastitis (infection of the milk ducts and breast tissue). Speak to your doctor if you develop either condition.

Know it takes time

Breastfeeding can be uncomfortable for the first few days, or longer for some women. But it eases with practise. If your nipples become cracked or sore, rub in leftover milk and leave to dry or treat with a breastfeeding and baby-friendly nipple cream. Also, make sure they are dry when you've finished feeding so they don't get chapped.

Avoid pacifiers for a few weeks

Don't give your baby a pacifier until after breastfeeding is well established (usually around four weeks), to avoid confusing her. Otherwise she may think she's feeding when she's sucking on a pacifier, which will affect how much breast milk she takes at a feed.

Be kind to yourself

Breastfeeding is a skill and it takes time and practise to become comfortable with it. Don't worry if you don't get the hang of it immediately, but make sure you ask for as much help as you need.

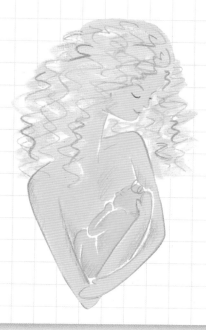

HOW TO BOTTLE-FEED YOUR BABY

Maybe you've tried breastfeeding, but it's not for you, or you want your partner to share the duties either with expressed milk or with formula. Whatever the reason, there's no need to feel guilty if you decide you want to bottle-feed—just enjoy the precious bonding opportunity. If you need help, talk to your baby's pediatrician.

○ **Know when to start**
If you're able to breastfeed and want to mix breast and bottle, most experts suggest waiting until your baby is three to six weeks old before trying a bottle. By then, breastfeeding is well established and the occasional bottle of expressed milk won't confuse her. However, if you leave it longer than three months to try mixed feeding you risk your baby rejecting the bottle. If you choose to give her formula, it's best to do it gradually, to allow your body time to adapt. Give the first few bottles when your baby is happy and relaxed—not when she's very hungry.

○ **Bottle buying**
There's no magic formula to finding a bottle your baby likes—it's a case of trial and error. Some babies will take to a particular shape, while others need features that ease wind or colic. Check the nipple, too—some are made to resemble the natural feel and shape of your breast, which could make the transition easier. Nipples come in slow, medium, or fast flow—start your newborn baby off with a slow nipple, and move to medium when she is used to the bottle. Never use a damaged nipple as it could be a choking hazard.

○ **Get into position**
Make sure you are sitting comfortably and look into your baby's eyes as you feed her. Hold your baby fairly upright for bottle feeds. Support her head so that she can breathe and swallow comfortably. Brush the nipple against your baby's lips and, when she opens her mouth wide, let her draw in the nipple. Give your baby plenty of time to feed. If you can, use skin-to-skin contact as you feed and switch arms halfway through, so she sees the world from both sides. Hold the bottle so that the nipple is always full of milk, otherwise your baby will take in air with her milk. Never leave a baby alone to feed with a propped-up bottle as she may choke on the milk. Your baby may need short breaks during the feed and may need to burp. When she's had enough milk (don't force her to finish the bottle), hold her upright and gently rub or pat her back to spit up any air (see page 18).

HOW TO MAKE UP A FORMULA BOTTLE

Making up your baby's bottle isn't simply a case of just mixing some formula with water—you need the right measurements, temperatures, and timings. Here's what you need to know.

○ **Keep it clean**
Wash your hands with antibacterial soap before touching any feeding equipment. This is an absolute must to avoid any nasty bacteria transferring from your hands to your baby's bottle. Make sure you clean and sanitize the bottles and nipples properly to get rid of any bugs (see page 22). As your baby's immune system is still developing, you'll need to keep her feeding kit super-clean by sanitizing it for at least the first six months.

○ **Get the temperature and the amount right**
Most local tap water is safe so pour the right amount into the bottle. Add the powder following the instructions on your formula packet. You don't want your baby to get too constipated or dehydrated, so use only the amount of powder that is recommended—no more and no less. You can also use bottled water or boil tap water for a minute, then cool it before using. Check that it's the right temperature by putting a few drops on your wrist; it should feel warm, never hot.

○ **Don't add any extras**
Whether or not the baby your baby is being weaned you should not add anything to the bottle (such as cereal). It won't mix well and won't do her tummy any good.

○ **Avoid the microwave**
The microwave should be a no-go area when it comes to your baby's food. Heating up the formula in this way may leave "hot spots" that burn your baby's mouth.

○ **Make fresh milk for each feed**
Although it's a bit of pain making bottles throughout the day, you should only make up enough formula for one bottle at a time. If need be, it's safe to keep prepared bottles in the refrigerator for up to 24 hours.

○ **Don't keep leftover milk**
If your baby doesn't drain the bottle then throw away the remains to avoid the risk of her having an upset stomach. Don't be tempted to save it for later.

HOW TO KEEP BOTTLES CLEAN AND SAFE

If you are bottle-feeding your baby—either with formula or expressed milk—it's important that you sanitize the bottles and nipples (and anything you use to prepare the bottles). Your baby's immune system is not as well developed as an older child's, so you need to sanitize anything that comes into contact with her mouth to eliminate bacteria that could make her ill.

○ **Wash everything in hot soapy water**
Make sure you clean any dried milk from the bottles; check the nipples carefully. Use a special bottle-brush to make sure you get into all the hard-to-reach areas. Many bottles are "dishwasher safe," but this won't remove all the dried-on milk so it's often easier to do it by hand.

○ **Sterilize your bottles before first use**
When you bring bottles home from the store, you'll want to sterilize them before giving them to your baby. Place all of the parts in a pot, cover them completely with water and bring the pot to a rolling boil. Boil for five minutes, then remove them .

○ **Use the dishwasher**
If your bottles are labeled as dishwasher safe, you can clean all of the parts on the top rack of the dishwasher, after any dried milk has been scrubbed off. Cleaning in a dishwasher with hot water and a heated dry cycle is an ideal way to get baby bottles clean. This kills more germs than simply washing the bottles by hand.

○ **Let bottles dry**
Place all of the pieces of feeding equipment on a special bottle-drying rack on your counter, or allow them to dry in the dishwasher. Do not use the pieces again until they have fully dried.

○ **Consider a sterilizer**
There are three main ways to sterilize bottles: boiling equipemnt in a pan; electric or microwave steamers (these use no chemicals only the heat from the steam to kill bacteria), or soaking in a chemicalsterilizing solution. Steam sterilizers are usually quick and efficient, with bottles ready in a few minutes. Always follow the instructions on the box. For the chemical sterilizing method, bottles and nipples are submerged in a special solution—usually made by dissolving a sterilizing tablet in cold water. They usually take a bit longer than steam sterilizing. Always follow the instructions on the pack.

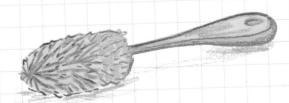

UNDERSTANDING NEWBORN SLEEP

You baby will sleep a lot in the first few weeks. For the first six weeks, you'll be at the mercy of her sleep patterns—it's tough, but remind yourself that she's adjusting to life and she needs to feed regularly too as her tummy is still tiny. A newborn baby can sleep for 18 hours a day in the first weeks and probably won't be able to stay awake for more than 45 minutes at a time, but this will gradually change.

HOW TO SWADDLE A BABY

Swaddling is when you wrap your baby in a thin cotton baby (swaddle) blanket from the shoulders down to help her settle (though some babies like to suck their fingers and prefer to be swaddled with their arms free). Never cover her face or head and don't wrap her too tightly as she needs enough room to be able to bend her legs. Check your baby frequently to make sure she is not overheating.

○ **Prepare your blanket**
Fold your swaddle blanket in half to create a triangle and place it on a soft, safe surface with the midpoint facing you.

○ **Position your baby**
Place your baby in the middle of the triangle,

Your baby might drop off mid-feed
Try and avoid the nap and snack routine where your baby doesn't take a full feed, then falls asleep. This can result in your baby having enough milk to stop hunger, but not to fill her up, meaning she'll wake more often. Try not to let her fall asleep while she's feeding and ideally put her down to sleep while she's awake.

She sleeps best in her own cot
Your baby's likely to nod off in all kinds of places, but always put her in her own crib. This is the safest place for your baby to sleep, both night and day, and experts recommend that you keep her crib in your bedroom for the first six months.

with her shoulders level with the long top side and feet facing the point (you).

○ **Tucking your baby in**
Holding her left arm close to her body, fold the right side of the blanket over her, pull carefully and tuck it under your baby's body. Repeat for the right side (reverse these instructions if you're left handed).

○ **Alternatively...**
You can also swaddle from the armpits down to leave her arms free, by laying your baby on the blanket so that the top is level with her armpits.

THE SAFE SLEEP RULES

Reduce the chance of Sudden Infant Death Syndrome, or SIDS (the sudden and unexpected death of a baby where no cause is found) by following safe sleep rules for babies. Full details from www.nichd.nih.gov/sts/

Don't

◯ Sleep on a sofa or in an armchair with your baby.

◯ Sleep in the same bed as your baby under any circumstances. If you feed your baby in your bed in the middle of the night, put her back when you're done.

◯ Allow your baby get too hot.

◯ Place any pillows, blankets, loose sheets, toys, or baby bumpers in the crib.

Do

◯ Always place your baby on her back to sleep with no covers or blankets at any time. For extra warmth, you can put your baby in footsie pajamas and/or a special baby sleep sack.

◯ Keep your baby away from cigarette smoke while you are pregnant and after birth. Keep your home, car, and other places your baby spends time, smoke free, and give up smoking if possible.

◯ Place your baby to sleep in a separate crib or bassinet in the same room as you for the first six months.

◯ Keep the room your baby sleeps in at a temperature of 61 to 68°F.

EXPERT TIP

NEWBORN SLEEP SECRETS TO TRY

• **Cluster breastfeed** In the latter part of the day, breast milk contains high levels of the hormone tryptophan, which aids the production of the sleep hormone melatonin. Try lots of feeds in the run up to bedtime to fill baby up and encourage the production of sleep hormones.

• **Background noise is OK** Light and noise do not bother newborn babies until around four to six weeks. Newborns can sleep through anything, so don't worry too much about noise.

• **Give white noise a try** You can buy CDs that mimic the noises inside the womb, but you need to use them quite early on.

TINA SOUTHWOOD
Sleep consultant

◯ A pacifier can reduce the risk of SIDS. If your baby uses one, don't place it on a string.

◯ Breastfeed your baby, if you can.

◯ Use a firm, flat mattress.

◯ Have your baby do Tummy Time often when she is awake, to strengthen her neck muscles. This may prevent her getting flat spots on her head too.

.... Questions you may be asking yourself ....

The first days after your baby is born can raise lots of questions in your mind.

"I'm coming to terms with a difficult birth experience—how can I deal with my feelings?"

The first thing to remember is that if anything traumatic or upsetting happened during your labor it was not your fault, and you're not alone. About 9 percent of women who give birth develop postpartum post-traumatic stress disorder (PTSD). An additional group of women may have some symptoms, including guilt, flashbacks, nightmares, bad memories, and feelings of anger. Many new moms find it hard to talk about and worry that their birth was difficult because they made the "wrong" choices, but this isn't true. It's possible to have a wonderful, empowering Cesarean section and a traumatic home birth, and vice versa. How you're treated can be a crucial factor. Feeling as if you're out of control, losing your privacy and dignity, fearing for your baby's safety and poor pain relief are just some of those factors. Counseling, such as cognitive behavioral therapy (CBT), accessed through your family doctor, can help alleviate anxiety. Postpartum International has information on its website how to find a support group in your area with other new moms who are with similar experiences. You can also ask your doctor for a referral to a psychiatrist, psychologist, or other mental health professional. PTSD stress disorder is a temporary, treatable condition.

"Am I producing enough breast milk?"

This is a common concern for many new moms, but try not to worry as, in all likelihood, you will produce exactly the right amount for your baby. Your breasts, regardless of their size, will always make milk as long as you breastfeed. At first you need to nurse a baby little and often, every couple of hours is perfectly normal. Newborn babies only have tiny tummies so it doesn't take much to fill them up. The volume of milk is not the only indicator of a good supply—if your baby is gaining weight, has lots of wet diapers and her poo is mustard yellow, then this is a clear indicator that she is more than likely getting all the milk she needs. After the first six weeks your breasts will not feel as "full" before a feed as they did at first because your body begins to establish effective supply and demand. So, when feeding your baby, listen to make sure she has a good latch and is swallowing properly. If you are expressing and are worried about milk supply, try to wait at least an hour post-feed before using your breast pump. You can also try alternating breasts; if you've fed your baby from your right breast, try expressing from the left. Always make sure you are well-hydrated, drink plenty of water throughout the day and when you are feeding. Remember, if your baby is struggling to latch on and you are concerned about her weight, do speak to your baby's pediatrician , who will be able to advise you further.

CHAPTER TWO
WEEKS ONE AND TWO

You are home with your newborn baby and he appears to spend most of his time eating, sleeping, and pooing. But he can do some amazing things already and there's much you can do to help him develop, even at this young age.

BE AMAZED AT HIS REFLEXES

Sucking is the first and most basic skill of all. When a newborn is placed at his mom's breast, he will usually try to latch on. This is a reflex, or involuntary action, along with his ability to grasp and make a fist (and grab your finger). So trust your instincts—listen to your baby and learn his responses. Sucking calms him, so let him suck his fingers if he wants to.

Your baby will be startled by sudden noises too, and it is normal for him to jump if he hears a loud noise. Babies are born with the Moro reflex (to encourage them to hold on to their mother), which can be triggered by sudden movement or a loud noise; he will cry and fling out his arms and legs. He will have this reflex until he's about six months old, so try swaddling to help him feel more secure at night, especially in the early days (see page 23). Play music, rub his back, and sing to him to soothe him.

RECOVERING FROM CHILDBIRTH

You are home, happy, proud, but also exhausted and sore. The first few days home with your new baby can be overwhelming and that tiny little bundle will demand a lot of your attention. So it's important not to forget about looking after yourself. You have been through a major physical and emotional experience and you need to give yourself the opportunity to get back on top form so you can be the best mom possible.

It's perfectly normal to find the transition to motherhood a struggle. You may worry you don't yet have the knowledge or skills to cope with a baby. Motherhood is a huge learning curve and you'll find your way as you go. These first few days will soon be a distant memory, but you'll find them easier to deal with if you prepare yourself.

Rest when you can

When it comes to sleep, you'll have heard that this can be the most challenging part of being a new mom. You need to adopt a new approach and doze when your baby does. Don't stay awake all day and expect to sleep all night; it won't happen. Instead, sleep in small chunks over a 24-hour period. If you can't sleep, just lie down on the sofa or in a dark room. Resting is almost as restorative as sleep. Or better still, once your baby is fed, have your partner to take him for a walk so you can get an uninterrupted doze. Lastly, ignore the ironing and don't do chores when your baby is sleeping. There's time for that later. For now, just rest.

Limit visitors

Everyone will want to come and see the new addition. To stay on top of numbers, keep it to family only for the first day or two. Give them a time to visit and a time limit. If that's not possible, and you are tired, ask your partner to entertain them while you have a lie down. Nobody will mind (and there's nothing wrong with staying in your pajamas either).

Accept all offers of help (and food) and ask visitors to bring you groceries when they come by.

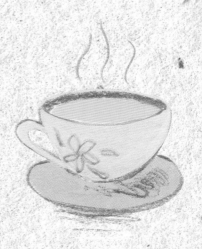

Your post-birth bump

When it comes to your body, it can be startling to look down at your post-birth self and realize that you still look pregnant; that's totally normal. You won't lose your bump overnight, or any time soon. Your uterus takes six weeks to contract to its non-pregnant size. Your abdominal muscles have also relaxed during pregnancy so everything looks fairly floppy. After six weeks you can start some gentle exercises—if your doctor says it's OK—but in the early days just relax and enjoy your new baby. Breastfeeding and sensible eating can help, but now is not the time to stress about a little mom tum.

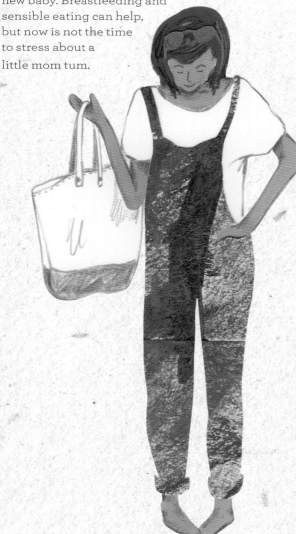

REAL LIFE

"Take a jug to the bathroom"

"When I had my baby, I did experience some tearing and had a few stitches as a result. Going to the loo made my stitches sting. My midwife suggested pouring warm water from a jug over myself as I was weeing. It was the best tip I've ever been given!"

ALISON, MOM TO SABINE, EIGHT MONTHS

If you have had stitches

If you needed stitches (more likely with first babies and less so with subsequent births), the good news is that the vast majority heal up quickly so they shouldn't bother you for long, and they're easily dealt with. The first 24 hours are often the worst and soreness goes after around two weeks. To help minimize discomfort drink plenty of water as it will sting less when you wee. Make sure you're eating lots of fibre, too, to prevent constipation. The first post-birth bowel movement can seem daunting, so make it as easy as possible, particularly if you've developed piles during pregnancy. If you become constipated ask your doctor for advice.

Some new mothers are reluctant to take painkillers, but the medication the hospital may prescribe for you to take home will ease the discomfort. The more comfortable you are, the better rested you'll be, and this also helps breastfeeding. If your stitches become more painful or soreness lasts longer than two weeks, you may have an infection so speak to your doctor. To boost healing, try pelvic floor exercises, as this increases blood flow to the area and speeds up healing. Keep the area clean and dry and wear cotton knickers. Change your maternity pad every two hours and occasionally leave your bottom half naked and lie on a towel to air the scar. Shower once or twice a day.

KNOW THE SPECTRUM OF POO

Depending on whether your baby's fed on breastmilk or formula, his poo will change as the days go by. After the first two or three days of meconium, drinking your breastmilk will cause your baby's poos to change to a lighter color. They will become bright or mustard yellow, loose and could possibly have a slightly sweet smell. He may poo during or after every feed, but this will settle down as his body gets into its own routine. Some breastfed babies only poo once every few days after the first few weeks but as long as your baby's stools are soft and are passed easily this shouldn't be a problem.

If you're formula feeding, your baby's poo will be thicker than a breastfed baby's and yellowish-brown in color.

EXPERT TIP

RIDING THE EMOTIONAL ROLLERCOASTER

When it comes to your mood, beware that, between two and five days after giving birth, you may have a day or so when everything feels too much (also known as the baby blues). It doesn't happen to everybody, but if it does it's very normal and very healthy. It results from a combination of hormonal changes following birth and tiredness. It can also be caused by a huge comedown after the elation of pregnancy, the drama of labor, and a rush of visitors. It's a healthy release, so don't stifle your tears; go with the flow and cry it out. Knowing that such an outpouring of emotion is to be expected should stop you worrying. However, if you're crying most days mention it to your doctor because it could be an early sign of postpartum depression (see page 52).

MIA SCOTLAND
Clinical psychologist

BASIC BABY CARE

So you've worked out how to change a diaper, feed, and dress your baby, but what else should you think about now you're home? Master the baby basics and keep your little one fresh and content.

Keep his skin soft and clean

As your little one's skin is so sensitive, the current advice is to bath your baby no more than two or three times a week, but give him a sponge bath every single day instead. This means cleaning his face and bottom with a washcloth or cotton balls and warm water.

With a separate ball of cotton ball for each eye, wipe once from the inner side to the outside, never rub backwards and forwards, as it can encourage infection. Moisten, then wring out a washcloth (so it isn't drippy) to wash the rest of your baby. Clean in the folds behind his neck and ears, too, because milk often gets trapped there. Using a separate bowl of water for hygiene reasons, do the same with his bottom area, lifting his legs up so you can get into all the creases. A new baby's skin is delicate and tends to dry out easily.

You can bath your baby in the kitchen sink, which is great as it's a comfortable height, or you can buy a baby bath. In terms of skin health, it's also a good idea not to use any perfumed products in the bath or indeed any lotions afterwards. Some of the chemicals in these products can trigger contact dermatitis, especially if there's a family history of skin problems or eczema.

Preventing diaper rash

When your baby is born, his skin will be very delicate and its protective barrier will not yet be fully formed. This means that diaper rash is a common problem, usually caused by irritation of the skin from prolonged skin contact with pee

and poo. The skin will look red and angry and if left in contact with the diaper may ulcerate, forming crusts. Diaper rash usually doesn't affect the skin creases at the top of the legs. To try and avoid the problem, change your baby's diapers frequently and never let him "sit" in a soiled one. You can also try a newborn-appropriate preventative diaper barrier cream

If he has diaper rash

If your baby does have diaper rash, use cotton balls and cooled, boiled water to carefully clean the area; baby wipes, particularly perfumed ones, can aggravate a sore bottom so are best avoided while the diaper rash persists. Then dry the area gently but thoroughly and apply a diaper cream that contains zinc oxide. This cream forms a protective barrier between your baby's skin and his diaper, and stops urine or faeces from coming into contact with your baby's sensitive skin. Some creams will also contain an antiseptic, which should help to soothe the area and prevent infection of the area.

As long as it's not too cold around the house, allowing your baby to have some "diaper off" at home time is also helpful for getting air to the area which will promote healing. Some moms

QUICK FIX

FIRST AID

Some parents find it useful to attend a baby first aid course (you can do this before you give birth), which can help prepare you in case of an emergency.

also find switching diaper brands can help (some brands are more absorbent than others so this makes sense). If you are using cloth diapers switching washing detergent can be helpful too; non-biological varieties are believed to be gentler for sensitive skin although there is no conclusive evidence of this.

If the rash still fails to clear up, or spreads to the creases in the groin then this may signal infection either with bacteria or fungus (candida), so see your doctor right away. He or she may prescribe an antifungal cream combined with a mild steroid, which should clear up the problem within a week. In some cases diaper rash may aggravate an underlying skin condition such as eczema in which case your doctor will advise you on how to manage this.

EXPERT TIP

CARING FOR THE UMBILICAL STUMP

After your baby is born, his umbilical cord will be clamped and cut, leaving 1¼ to 1½ inches of umbilical cord with a clip on the end. The clip will stay on for two or three days and may then be removed by a nurse. Whether the clip is removed or not, the remaining cord will gradually dry up, turn black and then fall off, which takes about seven to ten days. The scar will become your baby's belly button.

If you get the stump wet or give him a bath, that's fine, so long as you use plain water—avoid using any baby soaps, creams, or powders and pat the area dry afterwards.

Let the stump fall off naturally; don't pull it off yourself. Although very rare, belly button infections can develop during healing. Look out for redness, pinkish pus, and a different odour from usual, and talk to your baby's pediatrician about the best treatment.

DENYSE KIRKBY
Midwife

HOW TO BATH YOUR BABY

That first bath can be pretty nerve-wracking. Here's how to get confident—you'll soon both be looking forward to a wind-down bathtime.

○ **Get everything ready**
Make sure your bathroom is warm and have a towel, diaper, and pajamas ready before filling the bath. Pick a time when your baby isn't hungry or tired, so he's not irritable.

○ **Check the temperature**
Fill your baby bath with around 5 inches of water—enough to cover his chest. Put cold water in first then add hot; it should be 98°F, which is body temperature. Test with your elbow or wrist, these areas are more sensitive to heat than your hand. If you're unsure, use a thermometer.

○ **Wash his face and hair**
Undress your baby down to his diaper, place him on your knee and clean his face with a washcloth and the warm water. Wrap a towel around him and supporting him over the bath, wash his hair with plain water. Gently dry his hair then you can take off his diaper, wiping away any mess.

○ **Ease him into the water**
Lower your baby slowly into the water feet first, using one hand to hold his upper arm and support his head, neck, and shoulders on your arm. Don't let him go, hold him like this with his head out of the water until you are ready to bring him out again. Using your free hand, wash him gently with a sponge or washcloth. Never leave your baby alone.

○ **Go in order**
Wash your baby from top to bottom, front to back, to avoid spreading infections.

○ **Keep it simple**
It's best to bathe your newborn with just warm water for the first few weeks. As his skin is so delicate, using toiletries could leave it feeling dry or prone to irritation.

○ **Have fun**
Let him splash around in the water so he learns that bathtime is fun. When he is used to the bath opt for toys that allow you to sprinkle water on him—he'll love the sensation. Don't let him get cold; placing a warm flannel on his tummy can help.

○ **Wrap him up**
When you're done, lift him out of the water and immediately wrap him up in a warm, fluffy towel. Very gently, dry his head, and give him a cuddle so he warms up quickly.

○ **Dry him gently**
Gently pat him dry, paying particular attention to his bottom, any folds in his skin, and between fingers and toes, where dry, chapped skin is more likely to form.

○ **Join in**
Skin-to-skin contact is brilliant for bonding, so you or your partner can get in the bath, too. Just make sure you always dry and dress your baby first so that he does not get cold.

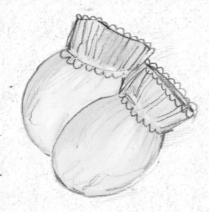

Treat nails with care

A new baby's nails are soft and flexible and they grow very fast. To stop your baby from scratching his face, put on some mittens or use socks. When it comes to trimming, use an emery board to file down the ragged edges. You can do this while your baby is feeding or sleeping.

Washing his hair

If your little one has lots of hair, you may want to wash it, but do it infrequently (once every couple of weeks) and choose a PH neutral shampoo, which is mild and un-perfumed, so there is no irritation to his scalp.

Give him a calming retreat

The less-is-more approach when it comes to his environment is also worth remembering. Newborns don't need lots of toys or mobiles as they can only focus about 10 to 12 inches. At this stage limit his stimulation rather than encouraging it. It's only after about four months that he may be able to focus on simple black and white images. Your face, with a loving expression, and your soothing voice tend to be the only stimulus your baby needs now. Keeping him calm will also encourage a better sleep pattern.

EXPERT TIP

DEVELOPMENT AND COMMUNICATING WITH YOUR BABY

Your baby will love looking at faces and if you stick out your tongue he could even stick out his tongue in response to copy you.

At birth his vision is still undeveloped. He can only fix on an object at 10 to 12 inches away, which is the perfect distance to study your face as you cradle him. Gently hold him, make plenty of eye contact, and talk to him in encouraging tones, calling him by name.

DR REBECCA CHICOT
Child development and parenting expert

Managing cradle cap

Dr Philippa Kaye explains, "Cradle cap, or seborrhoeic eczema, is the name given to the creamy yellow scales that often appear on a young baby's scalp. The skin can look greasy, flaky, and occasionally red. Cradle cap can spread behind the ears, onto the eyebrows and sometimes to other parts of the body.

"Cradle cap is very common and, however nasty it might look, it's usually harmless. It doesn't itch or cause your child any discomfort, it is not contagious and has nothing to do with hygiene. Cradle cap tends to affect babies in the first few months of life and is often at its worst during the initial weeks. The exact cause is not known, but it is thought to be related to an over-production of sebum, a fatty oil that moisturizes the skin. Experts suspect some babies have overactive sebaceous glands because they retain maternal hormones in their bloodstream after the birth. It's unclear why some babies are more prone than others, but we do know that most cases clear up once the oil glands are better developed.

"Mild cases of cradle cap usually clear up by themselves. To help it along, gently rub baby or olive oil into your baby's scalp and leave it overnight. In the morning, gently loosen the crust with a soft hairbrush and use a baby shampoo to wash the hair and scalp; don't pick at it as this could lead to it becoming infected. If the scales are thick they might not come off with just one treatment, so repeat the process over the next few days.

"If olive oil and baby shampoo doesn't work, you could try a specialist shampoo or cradle cap cream; ask your pharmacist for advice. See your baby'sif the cradle cap becomes infected (it will be red and inflamed) or you are concerned. Your baby's pediatrician might prescribe antibiotic or antifungal cream. A mild steroid cream might also be recommended it it's inflamed."

YOUR BABY'S CRYING

The sounds of your little one's cries are something you'll quickly become used to, but the reasons behind them aren't always easy to recognize. Your baby may not be able to talk, but he asks for what he wants through his cries. Working out what he's trying to tell you can be the key to keeping you both happy and calm. Don't panic and try different things until you work out the cause.

He's hungry

Hunger is one of the most common reasons why your baby cries, so this should be the first thing to consider. A new baby has such a tiny tummy that he can need hourly feeds, so it might seem like you've only just finished feeding him when he starts crying for more. This problem will fade as you settle into a routine as he grows.

He's uncomfortable

It might be that he needs burping if he hasn't settled after his feed or that he's in an uncomfortable position. Parents will start to learn the natural sound of their baby's cry. But when he's in pain it'll sound very different; it's more like a high-pitched shrill. Wind, colic (see page 48), and reflux (see page 36) can all also cause your baby discomfort, which results in excessive amounts of crying—speak to your doctor about the best way to treat them.

He needs changing

There's nothing like a soiled diaper to make your baby cry, so put this one up there as one of the first things to check. Looking down the back of his diaper is a quick way to work it out. Some will cry as soon as they dirty a diaper, others will wait a while before letting you know they need changing. Either way, at least these are easy tears to dry.

EXPERT TIP

EARLY SLEEP AND FEEDING PATTERNS
During the first months, your baby's sleep and bedtime habits change dramatically. If you have no problems feeding and your baby is healthy he will sleep for up to 18 hours a day in the first weeks, but he'll also continue to wake every few hours for a feed. Forget about strict routines and focus on establishing feeding, cuddling, diaper changing, and keeping him warm.

To establish a routine if you're breastfeeding, offer your baby the breast every few hours, whether or not he's asking for food. If he wants more, let him have more. Follow this pattern through the night as well so he takes regular feeds.

Let your baby have a long feed from one breast, then if he's sleepy, change his diaper. When he's alert again, offer the other breast. You're teaching him that this is a time for feeding, rather than a place to fall asleep.

TINA SOUTHWOOD
Sleep consultant

He's too tired
When a baby is overtired he is actually more likely to cry and fuss instead of falling asleep. A tired cry is normally very loud and cranky, but often fades away as he falls asleep. Try rocking him and making soothing noises as you settle him in his crib.

He wants a cuddle
In the first few weeks of your little one's life, he will want a lot of your attention, so enjoy lots of lovely skin-to-skin contact and try to interact with him as much as possible—this will help soothe him. All babies are different and some crave close contact with their parents more than others. Remember your new baby is used to being in the womb, so for the first few months of his life swaddling might also make him feel more secure (see page 23).

He's too hot or too cold
Check your baby's temperature. He might be trying to tell you that he's too hot or too cold. Newborns are more likely to cry when they're too cold as they're used to being warm and snuggled in the womb. That's why he may fuss when you're changing his diaper.

He's overstimulated
Babies are surprisingly good at picking up on tension, so those arguments that come with the stresses of being new parents might be the reason behind his tears. Or, he could simply need a break from all that passing around. We all need a little space sometimes, so just try to keep things calm and quiet while he calms down.

GETTING TO GRIPS WITH FEEDING

While some new moms and babies take to breastfeeding easily, there are lots of others who struggle. Many moms feel they don't get enough breastfeeding support in the early days. As a result they give up but feel terribly guilty about doing so. Here are some of the things you may encounter and tips to help.

A big, hungry baby

Big babies can have an insatiable appetite, which can feel physically and emotionally draining. The key with big babies is to feed as soon as possible. At the end of your pregnancy, your breasts have cells ready to make milk. If your baby has a feed after labor and you feed him often and on demand, your milk supply increases correspondingly; this can also get you through his growth spurts.

Baby has tongue-tie

Tongue-tie is caused by a tight or short frenulum, the membrane that attaches the tongue to the floor of the mouth. The frenulum should be thin and recede before birth. If this doesn't happen, tongue-tie occurs and movement of the tongue is restricted, which can make it difficult for your baby to latch on and suck freely when feeding, whether breast or bottle fed. Tongue-tie is more common in boys and can run in families, too. It can lead to poor weight gain, sore nipples, and lots of frustration. Tongue-tie usually resolves itself after about a year as your baby's tongue grows, but that won't really help with breastfeeding problems right now. If it's really affecting your feeding, talk to your baby's pediatrician; he or she may refer your baby to a surgeon for a frenulotomy. This involves a making small snip to separate the frenulum from the base of the mouth, sometimes with no anesthetic required.

Your baby is a grazer

Once the feeding frenzy of the first few weeks is over, most new moms hope their baby will settle into some sort of routine. However, some babies just graze round the clock for weeks and months on end, which can leave moms feeling frazzled. Some babies do this because their latch isn't great and they aren't getting enough at each feed; if you think this could be the case with yours talk to your doctor or make an appointment with a lactation consultant. Also, try to read your baby's cues. Is he actually hungry, or does he want a cuddle or even a nap? Get your partner to walk around with baby for a bit to see if he settles, as it may not be food he's crying for; if he can't smell your milk, he may not ask for it.

You have a baby with reflux (breast or bottle feeding)

Reflux is a fairly common condition and it occurs when your baby's milk comes back up into his food pipe or mouth. A baby's stomach contains acid, to help it digest food. Food that "comes back" is acidic, which can be painful for your baby if he vomits. Reflux usually eases off when you start weaning at around six months, and there are treatments that can help in the meantime. First, get a proper diagnosis from your baby's pediatrician. He or she may recommend an antacid-style medication for babies; this works very much like an indigestion pill for adults. Keeping your baby upright during and after feeds helps, as does feeding little and often, so let your baby feed frequently. A calming bath can soothe an upset tummy, too.

You've just had a Cesarean section

A Cesarean birth usually means longer recovery time for you and may impact on establishing breastfeeding if you're physically unable to sit and feed your baby, which can make it harder for baby to latch on. So try to breastfeed as soon as you're alert enough, in the recovery room if possible. Simply lying there, skin-to-skin, is often enough to prompt baby to nuzzle onto your breast and if you are drowsy, get your partner to hold him close to you.

When you can sit up, putting a rolled-up towel or small pillow across your lap can protect your incision. Use plenty of pillows to support the weight of the baby and to get him into a good position—some C-section women prefer lying on their side with the baby lying sideways to feed. Pain-relief medication can mask pain during feeding, making it easier.

Painful breasts

This is common. It's the first time your breasts and nipples will have been used in this way so tenderness is normal but outright agony needs to be addressed. Cracked and sore nipples can be a result of incorrect positioning.

It can help to try different feeding positions and to use the healing properties of breast milk itself—express a few drops and rub gently into your nipples, allowing them to dry naturally. Keep toiletries like shower gels away from nipples and air them as much as possible; cancel visitors for a few days and go top- and bra-less round the house. If you need to remove your baby from the breast because it hurts, break his suction by gently inserting your finger between his gums to avoid further damage.

Mastitis, from an infection in a milk duct, affects almost 10 per cent of breastfeeding women. It causes painfully swollen breasts and sometimes flu-like symptoms. If you develop mastitis, continue with regular feeds to keep your breasts as empty as possible. Make sure you rest and drink lots of water. If you continue to feel unwell, see your doctor as you may need antibiotics; these should be compatible with breastfeeding.

You're shy in public

Women have the legal right to breastfeed their babies in public in 49 states and the District of Columbia, but that doesn't stop some of us feeling self-conscious about it. Practise at home in front of a mirror, using clothes that drape over your breasts. Getting baby on the breast before he cries means you can feed without anyone noticing. There's also the two-vest top option: pull up the vest on top, then pull down the second vest underneath, to reveal only the breast for feeding. However, if you feel uncomfortable, then do what is best for you—if you prefer to feed in private then do so!

QUICK FIX

ENGORGED BREASTS

Try putting cold, raw, and washed Savoy cabbage leaves inside your bra (change it every two hours), to soothe your breasts.

Q&A

"How can I establish healthy feeding habits?"

Healthcare professional PENNY LAZELL says, "Whether you're going for breast or bottle, there are some things to think about when it comes to healthy feeding habits. The benefits of breastfeeding—even for the first weeks—are widespread. Aside from being free, the most immediate benefit is the bond that it creates between you and your baby. Breastmilk protects against all sorts of infections and diseases and your baby is less likely to suffer from diarrhea and vomiting, chest infections, and constipation.

"But not all new moms can or wish to breastfeed. If you use formula, that's your decision, because every mother, and every baby, is different. If the stress of breastfeeding or feeling uncomfortable with it is leaving you unhappy, then it could ultimately affect your baby. You need to give your little one lots of love and sustenance (breastmilk, formula, or a mixture of the two); that's all he needs.

"However you choose to feed your baby, it's important not to get hung up on times and amounts of feeds. If you're bottle-feeding, don't worry if your newborn is not drinking exactly the manufacturer's recommended amount every three hours. If he's happy and settled without finishing the bottle, then leave it (and throw it away). In the same way, if your baby is breast or bottle-fed and cries an hour after a feed, try feeding him again. Watching for your baby's hunger cries is important, too, especially if you're bottle-feeding as they take time to make. In the early weeks, cues can simply be a baby waking or fidgeting."

EXPRESSING YOUR MILK

Don't let the word "pump" deter you from giving it a go—expressing milk can help relieve your breasts if they are too full and uncomfortable, and a store of milk in the fridge or freezer allows you to get a good night's sleep while your partner does the 2am feed.

When to start expressing

Unless your baby was premature or is ill it's best to wait until your milk supply is established before starting to express. This is usually when he's around six to eight weeks. Express often—after the first feed of the day is a good time.

How to express

You can express by hand or with a breast pump or it can be a good idea to do a bit of both as the pump "sucks," but hands "milk"—the combination is similar to how your baby feeds. Expressing is a skill and may take a while to get the hang of, so relax before you start. Wash your hands thoroughly.

Hold a clean feeding bottle or container below your breast to catch the milk as it flows. To express by hand, cup your breast with the palm of your hand and walk your thumb up from your nipple until you feel a change in texture. Place your middle finger opposite your thumb and make a "C" shape and then start expressing—try to press back, bring together and press forward. Keep going until your milk flow subsides.

If you're using a pump, ensure all the washable parts are clean. With a manual pump, make sure the funnel isn't too small when your nipple is brought into the narrow part of the funnel, as this could be painful. Operate the handle as instructed on the packaging. If you prefer an electric pump, the motor will operate the pump for you. You should be able to alter the suction to suit you and just like the manual pump, make sure it fits you correctly.

It can take a while to get used to expressing, but it does get easier. It can take a couple of minutes

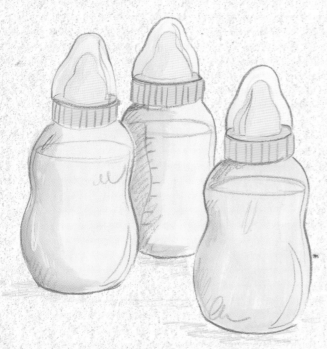

for your milk to start flowing. Pump as long as your milk is coming and swap breasts when your flow slows down (pump each breast twice).

Feeding expressed breastmilk

Your milk is best served fresh. But, if you're giving it to your baby after it has been in the fridge or freezer, there are some things to watch out for. Don't microwave expressed breastmilk as it will create dangerous hot spots that will burn your baby's mouth. If your baby prefers the milk at body temperature you can warm it in a bowl of lukewarm water.

If it's frozen, defrost it slowly by placing it in the fridge or try holding the container under cold running water. Don't shake the milk vigorously if it's separated, just gently swirl it. Defrosted milk can be refrigerated for up to 24 hours. Throw away any unfinished milk. Never refreeze breastmilk.

Storing breastmilk

Breast milk must always be stored in a clean container. It's a good idea to store expressed milk in small quantities to avoid waste and to warm or thaw quickly. Put the freshly expressed milk into clean feeding bottles with sealable lids, or in special breastmilk bags. Make a note of when you pumped the milk on each container. It will keep in a fridge for three to five days at 39°F or lower—buy a special thermometer if you are unsure of the temperature of your fridge. Alternatively you can freeze it for up to six months.

YOUR BABY'S WEIGHT

Your baby will be weighed at birth and again during his first week (at around four days). In the early days after birth, it's normal for babies to lose some weight (this is due to the fact that babies are being fed colostrum initially while waiting for the milk to "come in"). Your baby will be weighed by the nurse at the pediatrician's office to make sure he gets back up to his birth weight, and you'll be offered support if this doesn't happen. Unless you have concerns and request it, after the first week, your pediatrician's office will want to weigh your baby no more than once a month until he's six months of age, then no more than once every two months until he's a year old, and thereafter no more than once every three months.

Your baby's length may also be measured at intervals. His growth will be recorded on centile charts in his records (the charts show the pattern of growth that healthy children usually follow).

Medical records

Once your baby is born, the pediatrician's office will create a medical record for him. (Whether it's a paper file or a computerized record depends on how technologically advanced the doctor's office is. Either one will serve your child's purposes well.) The doctor will record all of your child's health information in the file and refer to it when treating your child. If a specialist needs to treat your child, then the pediatrician can send a copy of the file at your request. The pediatrician may offer you a vaccination card to bring to appointments to get updated with each immunization for your own records, if you so desire.

YOUR FIRST OUTING TOGETHER

This could be to visit the grandparents, Sunday lunch with friends or just a trip to the park. Whatever the event, when it's time to leave the doona on the sofa, have a shower, and head out with your baby, here's what to think about.

○ **Be realistic about timings**
Give yourself lots of time and make sure you have everything you need. Schedule outings for any time that suits you and don't be ambitious—a walk or coffee is fine. Have a couple of goes at putting up the pram or stroller or using the baby carrier, so you know how to use them. You'll look like a pro and won't have any last minute panics.

○ **A helping hand**
If you need support, you could ask someone to help. From pushing the pram to holding your handbag while you search for a diaper mat, another pair of hands is useful.

○ **Essentials to pack**
Pack a diaper bag with diapers, wipes, a spare one-piece, and anything you need for feeding. Have essentials such as your wallet in front pockets and bring a drink and snacks for you to keep up your energy up.

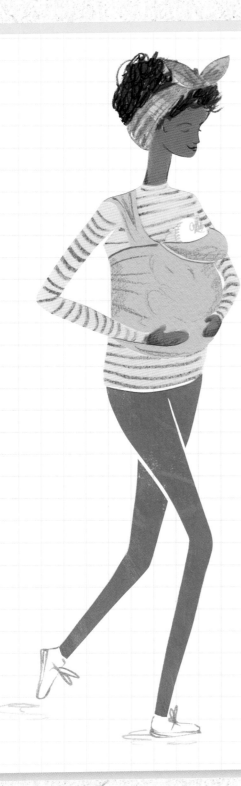

Prepare your baby when you're ready to go
Don't get your baby ready until the last minute, when your bag is packed, the pram ready or your car seat is in place. It's a good idea to give him a feed and change his diaper before you leave the house.

Dress him in appropriate layers
Avoid dressing your baby in bulky, tight clothes; opt for layers you can add or remove if he is too hot or too cold. If you're outside, a cotton hat will keep him warm, as he'll lose and retain most heat through his head. Unfasten his coat when you go into a shop, so he doesn't get too hot.

Don't rush
If you need to leave your house later than expected to fit in a feed, do it. Everyone (especially mommy friends) will understand. And it's better to be 15 minutes late than have an unhappy, crying baby and a stressed-out you.

Offer comfort in unfamiliar places
Keep making eye contact and talking to your baby while you push or carry him.

Enjoy yourself
Remember, this is a brilliant opportunity for you to socialize too, whether it's with friends in a restaurant or baby-mesmerized random people in the street.

Don't panic...
If the first trip still doesn't go to plan, don't see it as failure. Just try again tomorrow.

When should you go back to work?

This an issue that can leave many moms in a dilemma. The answer is when it feels right: it could be any time from six weeks old or at least three months old. It's your decision and whatever conclusion you come to will be the right choice for you.

Your emotional needs

This should be your first consideration. It's very easy to say goodbye to your work colleagues when you go on maternity leave cheerily promising to see them in three

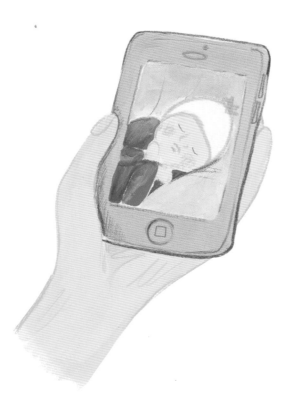

months time, only to discover that being away from your baby is going to be harder than you thought. Talk to your partner about how you feel as this will affect your start date. You may equally be climbing the walls at the loss of conversations that don't involve poo color.

Think about finances

There are ways to save money by cutting back on things like cable TV, cell phone data plans, expensive haircuts, and more. When you consider going back to work, think about how much money you will earn after taxes and how much you'll be paying for childcare.

Feeling out of the loop

Some moms worry about being out of the work place for an extended period and are concerned about the effect this might have on their career. You might consider picking a slow workday to visit the office with your baby in tow to introduce him to everyone. You'll get to catch up with everyone in person and see what's new in the office.

Sorting childcare

Sorting out who will care for your baby is going to have a bearing on when you end your maternity leave and return to work (see page 74). If you want or need to return to work but you're not ready for your baby to be looked after by someone outside the family, consider having your husband take time off. If he can't use his paid vacation or sick days, he may be eligible for the Family and Medical Leave.

NOTES

CONGRATULATIONS—YOU'VE MADE
IT THROUGH THE FIRST WEEKS AND ARE
SETTLING INTO YOUR NEW LIFE AS A MOM!

CHAPTER THREE
WEEKS THREE AND FOUR

Bonding with your little one is vital for her health and wellbeing, not to mention your happiness as parents. It's something we expect to be immediate like an animal instinct. But, like the start of any relationship, it can take a bit of work to get going.

COMMUNICATING WITH YOUR BABY

Any time between now and seven or eight weeks, your baby will start to smile. Smile back, make different faces, and be curious about what your baby is trying to tell you. While a smile might be the first enjoyable marker of communication, your baby will have been "talking" to you since birth.

Bonding is something we expect to kick in at first sight. For some it does, but for many it takes time (and effort). The effort is, of course, well worth it. Your baby needs a loving relationship to develop emotionally and physically. The environment outside the womb is very different to inside, and that can cause anxiety for her. Good bonding helps overcome this, and there are a few simple ways to help you feel that connection.

In the first four to six weeks, your newborn needs little to stimulate her, but what she does need is you. Some experts refer to this post-delivery period as the fourth trimester, as babies still crave the environment of the womb. Lots of skin-to-skin contact is very important, especially if she is bit colicky or fractious (see page 48). If she is having a problem settling, take her into a dark, quiet room, hold her, rock her, sing her a lullaby, play some white noise (to mimic the rushing noise inside the womb), and try to soothe her to sleep.

Consistency of care

This doesn't mean you need a strict routine, just that the people who care for your baby—for example, you and your partner—should always be there for her in the first weeks. Babies get to know the style of the person looking after them and find this reassuring. Research also suggests that being attended to in the same way by the same person, builds connections in your baby's brain and helps reduce stress.

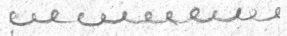

EXPERT TIP

WHY SKIN-TO-SKIN CONTACT HELPS

Make time for cuddles, especially skin-to-skin contact. This so-called kangaroo care helps regulate your baby's breathing and temperature and makes your baby feel calm. Lots of this cuddling releases the bonding hormone oxytocin in both moms and dads. This is the beginning of a life-long bonding process between parent and child and it's a great way for new dads to bond with their new baby too.

DR REBECCA CHICOT
Child development and parenting expert

Responding to her needs

Reacting to your baby is key to making her feel secure. This could be recognizing that she's hungry and feeding her, or even the simple act of changing her diaper when she needs it. The good old "mother's instinct" or "attachment" as psychologists call it, means your baby learns that she can rely on you.

Get talking to your baby

The sound of your voice will remind your baby of her time in the womb. She'll recognize the rhythm of your voice, and probably that of your partner or any other person you talked to a lot too. Communicating with your baby also demonstrates that you are listening to her, further building her trust in you.

Patience

Finally, be patient about the developing bond. If you're not feeling an instant rush of love for your baby, don't stress. Bonding can sometimes take a few weeks, and the more traumatic a birth you had, the bigger impact this can have on the process. If it has been a few weeks, and you still find it hard to connect with your baby, then it's worth talking to your doctor or therapist to rule out postpartum depression (PPD). Rest assured, the bond will eventually form and is worth the wait.

DRESSING YOUR BABY

When you are heading outside with your baby in tow, you need to ensure she's dressed properly so she stays cosy and warm on cold days without overheating, or cool and comfortable in warmer weather.

When it comes to dressing babies (and toddlers), layering is key. Wrapping your little one up in several layers means that not only can you ensure she is warm enough, but you can easily remove a layer to prevent her from overheating. Starting off with a good-quality base layer helps to regulate temperature and draw moisture away from your child's skin. Go for cotton T-shirts with snaps, long-sleeved one-pieces, or top-and-trouser sets,

and cardigans. Padded one-pieces are great for going out when it is cold. Consider how easy it will be to put on and take off your baby; a full-length front opening makes diaper changes or undressing a sleeping child much easier. Also bear in mind comfort-focussed features such as zip garages (special zip catch covers), so your baby can't scratch herself, or soft linings that are gentle against her sensitive skin.

Later down the line, when it comes to choosing outerwear for older children, look out for details such as reflectors or detachable hoods that prevent them becoming caught on things.

READY FOR TUMMY TIME?

It may be around now that your baby is ready for "tummy time," which involves lying her on her tummy on the floor, on a clean sheet or play mat

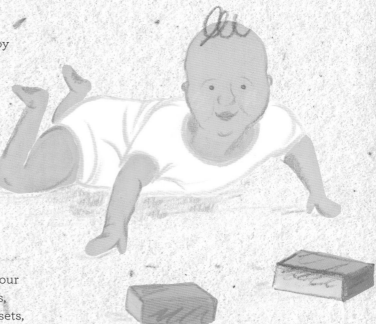

when she is fully awake. Tummy time is a great way to help develop your baby's fine and gross motor skills. It's the start of her being able to push herself up, learn to roll over, sit up, crawl, and eventually stand. It allows your baby to improve, exercise, and strengthen her neck control, which is fairly floppy when she's a newborn. It also helps improve your baby's orientation skills as it gives her a different view of the world.

Spending time on her tummy can also help treat flat-head syndrome that can result from laying on her back all the time as it takes the pressure off the back of her head, giving it a chance to round off. Tummy time is also a brilliant way to bond with your baby and gives you time to play together. While your baby may not love it at first, it won't be long until she enjoys her new view of the world. Start tummy time with your baby as soon as you feel she's ready.

Tummy time is not for sleeping though—always put her down to sleep on her back.

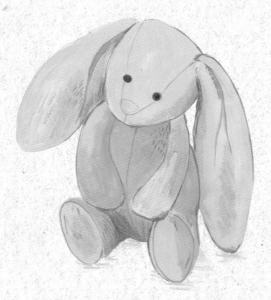

EXPERT TIP

INTRODUCING TUMMY TIME

Some babies get distressed the first few times they lie on their stomachs, so make sure she's happy, fed, and changed before you begin. Try anything from 15 seconds to two minutes a few times a day—any amount, no matter how brief, is beneficial. Start with short periods when she's a few weeks old and build it up to 20 minutes a day (broken down into short periods throughout the day) by the time she's three to four months. Pop her on a baby blanket on the floor—not on the sofa in case she rolls off. If she's very young (a few weeks old) and struggling to hold her head up, gently turn her head to one side so she doesn't struggle to breathe. Stay with her the entire time she's on her tummy in case she's unable to hold her head up. Lie beside her so she can see you. If she does become unhappy, try waving a toy in her eye line. If she really doesn't like it, try placing her upper body and arms over a nursing pillow for support.

PENNY LAZELL
Healthcare professional

BEGINNING TO SOCIALIZE WITH YOUR BABY

It's official. Becoming a mom doesn't mean you have to say goodbye to a social life. In fact, your baby may be your ticket to lots of new friendships. One little-mentioned benefit of new motherhood is that it is a great opportunity to expand your social circle. Whether that's making new friends or engaging with your current ones in a new way, there are super simple ways to connect.

If you're the first of your friends to have a baby, keeping in touch with women you met at your prenatal classes is a great way to bring some mom friends in your life. You'll be able to compare what you're going through and indulge in a gossip. Get time in for coffee. Meeting up with other new moms with your babies is really more for you at this stage; it gives you a chance to have a catch up while your babies take in the outside world.

Try baby groups

Your baby's pediatrician may know of local baby groups you can try. Libraries have baby-reading groups and your local gym may have swimming or baby yoga classes, which is another place to meet other moms (and amuse your baby). Have a look online too. Strike up a conversation with moms you meet in the park. Be open about your experiences of motherhood too as it will make other moms feel comfortable opening up to you.

Keep up with old friends

If none of your old friends have babies, don't forget them. Maintaining these friendships can help you keep your sense of identity. Some may naturally fade after a while, but good friends will still want to hang out with you and play auntie to your new addition.

WHAT IS COLIC?

Colic is a condition characterized by your baby crying or appearing distressed for long periods of time, several times a day, for no obvious reason. On top of inconsolable crying, a colicky baby may also arch her back, draw her legs up to her tummy, become stiff, pass wind, and clench her fists. Colic affects about one in five babies, usually starting in the first month, and can extend to the six-month mark. Even though it's usually harmless for your baby, the constant crying can really take its toll on you.

What causes colic is still uncertain, but the first thing to do is rule out wind caused by your baby gulping down too much air. If your baby gulps down her feeds, check she's latched on and positioned properly. If you're using a bottle, you could try anti-colic nipples (so she swallows less air when she's feeding).

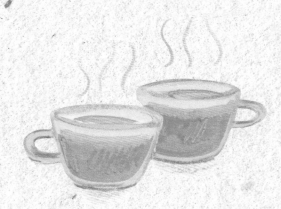

Q&A

"I think my baby has colic. What can I do?"

Healthcare professional PENNY LAZELL says, "A baby who swallows air may also need regular burping during her feeds. Another issue is that she may have a temporary intolerance to lactose in breastmilk or cow's milk protein in formula. All that may be needed is for her gut to mature a little more. Formula-fed babies may improve on a formula with reduced or no lactose—but only do this under the advice of your baby's pediatrician. If you're breastfeeding you could try following a special lactose-free diet for a fortnight (again talk to the pediatrician first). Many moms find cutting out coffee helps, too, as caffeine passes through to breastmilk, potentially aggravating symptoms.

"If you are breastfeeding, you can make some changes to your own diet, with hopes that the absence of certain potentially problematic ingredients in your breast milk may positively affect your baby's colic. Consider eliminating any or all of these items from your menu, for the time being: dairy products, caffeine, cabbage, onions, or anything else that you think could be triggering it.

But intestinal problems aren't the only issue. Some babies are more sensitive than others, and over-stimulation (such as picking them up and putting them down constantly) may cause colic. In addition, a traumatic delivery may have an influence, and there's also evidence that smoking in pregnancy doubles the chance of your baby developing colic.

"You can try comforting her by holding, dancing, or walking around with her. She may relax with some skin-to-skin contact in the bath. Alternatively, a fussy baby may find being picked up too often distressing. See if your baby is calmer if put in her cot in a darkened room.

"The good news is that colic always improves on its own, so medical treatment isn't usually necessary. However, there are some over-the-counter treatments that contain simethicone drops or lactase, which may be effective. But, only ever make these changes under the guidance of your baby's pediatrician."

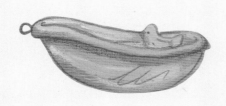

REAL LIFE

"How I helped my baby with colic"

"Sam was three weeks old when he'd cry for most of the day and night, clench his fists, and pull his knees up to his chest or kick vigorously as if he was in constant pain. He didn't sleep, his face would be bright red from crying, and each feed seemed to make him uncomfortable. The only way I could get him to sleep would be to take him for a drive in the car or a walk in his stroller. The pediatrician recommended infant indigestion medication and suggested buying anti-colic bottles, which really helped. We also introduced a bath every night to relax his tummy. Dealing with colic is so hard, but it does get better with time."

ELLIE, MOM TO SAM, FOUR MONTHS

STAYING ENERGIZED FOR BREASTFEEDING

It's vital to keep your energy levels up with nutritious meals and snacks and lots of fluids when you are breastfeeding. Your body is working hard to produce milk, so you're going to need all the energy you can get as breastfeeding burns extra calories on top of your daily needs; you should be eating an extra 500 to 600 kcal per day.

The same healthy eating guidelines apply to breastfeeding moms as to other women. Breastfeeding mothers can feel hungry quite often, which is perfectly normal. So in addition to eating balanced meals, you'll need to snack through the day on these healthy choices.

Starchy carbs
You need starchy carbohydrates to keep your energy levels up. Pick potatoes, rice, or pasta, but go for whole grain or wholewheat versions, as they'll keep your digestive system healthy. You could have a small pot of potato salad, a slice of wholemeal toast with a sliced banana, or a small portion of brown rice salad.

Fresh fruit
For on-the-go snacks, you can't beat fresh fruit. Bananas are the ultimate portable snack as they just need peeling and you can eat them straight away, but apples, satsumas, or a small bunch of grapes will also give you an energy and nutrient boost.

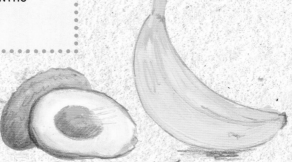

Eat fish

Nutrients from fish, such as omega-3 fatty acids, are passed onto your baby through your breast milk, so including regular portions is good for you both. Eat 8 to 12oz of low-mercury fish per week. Try tuna salad on toast or crackers for a quick-and-easy snack.

Snack on vegetables

Make up snack pots of carrots or sliced capsicums and eat with a few spoonfuls of houmous. Sliced cucumber is great because it has a high water content, so it's perfect for rehydrating you while you breastfeed. You could also try a small bowl of vegetable soup, which will fill you up and keep you going for a few hours.

Go for protein

Boost your protein intake and keep youself feeling fuller for longer with a small portion of eggs or meat. You can buy small packs of cooked chicken, which is great as a snack on its own, or in a sandwich.

Don't forget dairy

Aim for at least two servings of dairy per day. Go for a glass of milk—perfect for having with you when you sit down for a feed, or try a chunk of cheese. You could also have a pot of yogurt, but watch out for varieties that are very high in sugar.

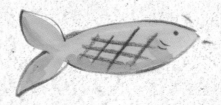

Nuts and seeds

An excellent source of protein and essential fatty acids, nuts and seeds are an ideal snack as you can keep a handful of them in your bag when you're out and about.

Dried fruit

Rich in iron, dried fruit is a great snack to have to hand when breastfeeding. Try raisins, prunes, or apricots.

Keep up your fluid intake

Fluids are extremely important when you're breastfeeding as you are, of course, giving up so much each time you feed. It's recommended that breastfeeding women drink 25fl oz extra per day, which is about four more glasses than you would normally drink. Make sure you always have a drink beside you when you are breastfeeding. Water, milk, and unsweetened fruit juice are good options to choose. Remember though, your baby's intestinal tract is immature so if you have consumed large amounts of citrus fruits or juice she may be sensitive to it. If she's unusually windy or uncomfortable, try cutting back. But always consult your baby's pediatrician if you have any concerns about her health.

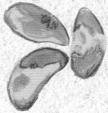
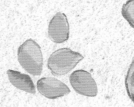

QUICK FIX

BREASTFEEDING

Try drinking fennel tea—a study in the Journal of Clinical Nutrition found it could help aid milk supply.

Q&A

"I am concerned about PPD, what should I do?"

"Never feel guilty for asking for support—whether from friends, family, or your doctor. There are some support groups that have helplines and many produce leaflets and run phone (sometimes text) lines (see Resources page 155). They also often provide advice for partners or family about supporting a loved one, too. While the people on the other end of the phone line often aren't health professionals, they do have training and can support, listen, and help you find the right advice."

DID YOU KNOW?

Clinical psychologist, Mia Scotland says, "Postpartum depression can also be missed because the mom loves her baby fiercely. It's a myth that all people with the condition struggle to love their baby."

BE AWARE OF POSTPARTUM DEPRESSION

New parenthood can be incredibly overwhelming, and postpartum depression (PPD) symptoms can start soon after giving birth and last for months or longer. In the hectic, sleep-deprived chaos of caring for a newborn, PPD can be missed or ignored. But with so many moms suffering from the condition and effective treatments available, never feel ashamed to seek help.

PPD can interfere with your day-to-day life and can be associated with increased anxiety. Some women feel they're unable to look after their baby, or they feel too anxious to leave the house or keep in touch with friends.

It is often missed because health professionals don't know how you're feeling or moms try to hide their condition for fear they'll be judged. But treatment will help both your health and the healthy development of your baby, as well as your other important relationships. Seeking help for postpartum depression does not mean you're a bad mother or that you're unable to cope. It's time to take care of yourself, so see your doctor if you have any of the following symptoms:

Low mood
It's normal to feel baby blues in the first few days after giving birth, but most women start to feel more positive after a week or two. For women with PPD, feelings of sadness or irritability persist.

Apathy
If you have PPD, you may also lose interest in the world and find it hard to take part in activities or motivate yourself.

A lack of energy
Of course, having a baby can be very tiring and this is normal, however PPD can also cause a general feeling of constant tiredness or fatigue.

Sleep problems

The exhaustion of looking after a baby who won't sleep or who wakes often can make PPD worse, but you may also find that you struggle to get to sleep or wake in the night.

Lack of confidence

Sufferers can start to question their decisions and have difficulties with concentration.

Feelings of guilt or self blame

Postpartum depression can make you feel very anxious even when the baby is happy and thriving.

A change in appetite

Losing your appetite and interest in food can be a sign that you may have PPD. But so can comfort eating to try and make you feel better.

Feelings of guilt

You may experience feelings of self-blame.

Frightening thoughts

Some women who have PPD get thoughts about harming their baby or themselves. These thoughts, known as obsessional ruminations, are very rarely acted upon. If you're troubled, discuss it with your family doctor who may refer you for help.

POSTPARTUM PSYCHOSIS

Postpartum psychosis is a rarer and more serious mental health condition that can develop after giving birth. It's thought to affect around one in 1,000 women. Possible indicatins include bipolar-like symptoms or hallucinations, and the condition is regarded as a medical emergency.

Seek immediate medical help if you think you or someone you know may have developed postpartum psychosis. If you think there's a danger of imminent harm to you, your partner, or your baby, you should call 911 or go to the Emergency room and ask for help.

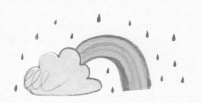

REAL LIFE

"I couldn't stop worrying"

"Around a month after my baby was born I felt I was having difficulty bonding with her and was crying frequently for no reason. Despite the fact she was well looked after, and the pediatrician was happy she was healthy and thriving, I couldn't stop worrying about her and my abilities as a mom. It was weeks before my partner noticed something wasn't quite right and he persuaded me to see my family doctor and talk about it.

"My doctor was really understanding. She gave me lots of advice (which included recommending taking up some regular exercise) and offered to refer me to a counselor. She also recommended a self help group in my area. There is lots of help out there and I'm so glad I talked to someone rather than bottling up my feelings."

ANONYMOUS

Using your support network

Being a new mom is undoubtedly an incredible experience, but it can be tough on your body and emotions. Remember, you're not alone—so be open to the people who can help you.

Your partner

When it comes to your partner, the support is both emotional and practical (or at least it should be). Your loved ones are always brilliant to lean on as they know you best. OK, so he may not be able to instinctively understand certain things, such as what it's like to breastfeed (or struggle with it), but he can learn. Help get him clued up by taking him along to some support groups or by suggesting that he talks to the experts as well. This may help him be there for you. You're a team, so make sure you work like one. No partner? Lean on good friends and family members—they will want to support you and can be invaluable as they know you best.

Your family doctor

Your doctor will have become a familiar face by now and should be your first port of call if you have any medical worries that need attention for yourself during this transitional time. Don't feel nervous about making appointments to dicsuss anything you're concerned about.

Your baby's pediatriacian

Your baby's pediatrician has been looking after your newborn since the beginning. In the early days of your life as a mom, his or her job is to make sure that your newborn is healthy and happy and that breastfeeding is going well. The pediatrician's advice can be invaluable.

Lactation consultant

Need some health with breastfeeding as a new mom? A lactation consultant is the person to call—she is specially trained to help you and your baby perfect your latch and make breastfeeding comfortable and second-nature for both of you. Your lactation consultant may visit you at home, meet you at a local destination, or even Skype/ Facetime with you on the computer. Depending on your needs, she may meet with you only once or follow up several times, until you've got the hang of things. She may also recommend local mother-and-baby breastfeeding groups.

Your baby's grandparents

They've been there and done it all—so whether you're close or have a trickier relationship—the support of grandparents can be amazing. If they live nearby, grandparents may help babysit, or just make that much-needed cup of coffee or meal.

Don't forget your friends

Good friends are to be valued and when you become a mom you'll find out just how brilliant they can be. The "already-a-mom" friend is often the most vital because she can reassure you, share advice or swap stories. More practically, friends who live locally can help if you have a logistical emergency. The wider your network the easier it is to find someone who can help out at any given time.

Postnatal baby groups

There are plenty of groups you can attend to meet moms in a relaxed and informal setting and share your concerns. When it comes to breastfeeding, look for your local chapter of La Leche League, or search online for a moms' meetup group, where leaders or moms can advise you on different positions to try that you may not have thought of.

Look online

Fire up your laptop, log onto the internet, and you'll instantly have tons of information at your fingertips—no matter what time of day or night it is. The internet is packed with sites that can be really helpful—just ensure you look at trusted websites such as www.healthychildren.org or www.motherandbaby.co.uk

Helplines

While the internet is fantastic, it can feel impersonal. Sometimes having a chat with a human (rather than a screen) can be a brilliant option. Occasionally we all need to speak to someone who doesn't know us and who won't judge us on any level. We have given you some ideas in the Resources section at the back of the book (see page 155).

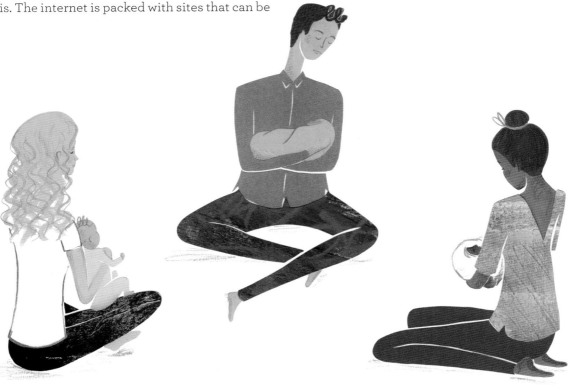

CHAPTER FOUR
BY SIX WEEKS

By this stage your baby needs milk every three to four hours during the day. You'll need to be more flexible in the evenings when he can get hungry, and give him milk at night if he wants it, but you don't need to wake him up to feed him. He'll want to nap approximately every hour during the day.

HAVE FUN TOGETHER

Your baby will be becoming more alert now. Any time between one and three months he will start to lift his head. This is the precursor to having strong enough neck muscles to fully support his head. Give your baby regular tummy time on a play mat on the floor (see page 46) while you also talk and smile to him.

If he is having a problem settling to sleep, take him into a dark, quiet room, hold him, rock him, sing him a lullaby, play some white noise (to mimic the rushing noise inside the womb), and try to soothe him to sleep. After six weeks, you could consider buying a little projector light that plays soothing images and womb sounds or the sounds of the ocean (white noise), although this may not work well for sensitive babies.

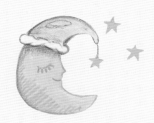

REAL LIFE

"I thought I'd never sleep again"

"When I had Harry, he only slept for two hours at a time, day and night. I felt stuck in an endless sleep/eat cycle that left me exhausted. Of course, getting into a better routine helped and eventually, he slept through the night just before he was a year old. I know the difficult times feel like they last forever, but it's important to remember, you will get a good night's sleep again one day."
CATHERINE, MOM TO ANNA, FOUR MONTHS AND HARRY, FIVE

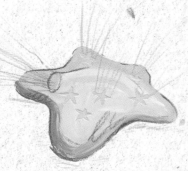

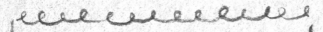

EXPERT TIP

ESTABLISH A LOOSE ROUTINE

Between now and three months, babies are more alert and risk becoming overtired. This is a key age to focus on sleeping patterns. Your baby needs 16 to 18 hours sleep, but may start fighting it.

When your baby wakes in the day, change, feed, and wind him, then play. This will take almost an hour and he'll start to tire again; he may stop making eye contact, arch his back, and move his head from side to side. Put him into his bed, tell him it's sleepy time, and leave him to drift off. At this age don't leave him to grizzle for more than five minutes, so if he doesn't settle, try playing white noise, rocking the crib, or singing a lullaby.

Demonstrate to your baby the difference between night and day. At night, keep the lights low, and don't interact while you feed him. Keep it boring and he'll learn that daytime is for activity and night is for sleeping.

TINA SOUTHWOOD
Sleep consultant

BABY MASSAGE

Massage is a great baby calmer and can help your bond to grow stronger. What's more, it's pretty easy once you know what to do. While any one-on-one time with your newborn is important, baby massage comes with extra benefits.

Touch produces the nurturing hormone oxytocin, which is great for bonding, as well as promoting sleep. Baby massage could also help relieve discomfort from colic or constipation.

Try a class

It's a good idea to enrol in a class to see how it's done—and attending classes will become easier as the weeks go by and your baby stays awake for longer periods. If you don't go to a class, invest in a book to ensure you have the correct technique. For example, never massage a newborn's head, as it's still developing. Also, avoid putting pressure on joints.

When you get started...

Choose the right time—your newborn may be in the mood for a massage around 45 minutes after a nap and feed. When all his needs have been met, he'll probably be in a "quiet-alert" period. But remember, babies have good and bad days, so if he starts crying, stop, give him a cuddle and just try again later or another day.

Make it soothing

Dim the lights and create a relaxing atmosphere. Place a towel on a diaper mat or on the floor in a warm room, undress your baby, and lay him on his back, facing you. When it comes to products, try organic sunflower seed oil designed for baby massage.

YOUR POSTNATAL CHECK-UP

Although it is generally called the six-week check-up, your first post-birth doctor's appointment might actually take place any time between six and eight weeks after your baby's birth. It's a time when your OB/GYN will make sure you're coping OK with parenthood and recovering from the birth well. It's the perfect opportunity for your family doctor and your baby to meet if they haven't already.

Every doctor will handle this check-up differently and time limitations can mean you'll feel all of your issues haven't been addressed. So write down any questions you want to ask (as and when you remember them) and don't be afraid to get out the list when you get there—even if it seems rather long. Before you leave the surgery give your list a quick once-over to make sure you haven't missed anything.

How to book your six-week check-up

Your doctor should remind you toward the end of your pregnancy, or at the hospital, to call the office to schedule an appointment once your baby is born. While a standard ten-minute appointment is the normal length you'll be given, you can ask for a longer session if you think that won't be long enough to address all of your concerns.

It is important not to see this session as a one off. It is part of an on-going relationship that you and your baby build up with your doctor over time.

What could happen at your check-up

Your doctor will carry out various checks to assess your general health and recovery from the birth, as well as how you are coping as a mom. Your doctor may:

○ Test your urine to make sure your kidneys are working as they should and that you haven't got an infection.

○ Weigh you.

○ Check your blood pressure.

○ Check any stitches you had after the baby's birth, either vaginally or following a C-section, to make sure they've healed.

○ Ask you if you're still experiencing any lochia (normal discharge after giving birth) and whether you've had a period since your baby's birth.

○ Check that your uterus has returned to its pre-pregnancy size, shape, and location, and that your cervix is following suit.

Questions your doctor may ask you

As well as the physical examination, your doctor will talk to you about your emotional wellbeing. He or she may talk to you about booking a smear test if you haven't had one in the last three years and will discuss your contraception options.

Be honest with your doctor about any problems you're having. Tell him or her if you're feeling really low and overwhelmed, aren't sure about something or you constantly need the loo. The more the doctor knows, the more he or she will be able to help you, or refer you for an appointment with a specialist if necessary.

Your sex life now

Babies change everything—your sleep, body, daily routine, even your relationship. But what very few new parents talk about is the impact they have on your sex life. Aside from your body having been stretched and pulled about, a new baby's needs are so overwhelming and exhausting that sex, naturally, becomes a low priority. When it does resume though, post-baby sex can feel different in a positive, exciting way. So, while you may think your days of wild sex are over, new parenthood can in fact improve on where you left off.

Depending on the birth, it can take weeks or months to feel like you want penetrative sex again. You can feel anxious about lots of things: is your vagina looser because of the birth, tighter from stitches, too dry (which can happen if you're breastfeeding), or just whether sex will hurt. The truth is sex after a baby can feel different, but not necessarily in a negative way. If you've had a Cesarean section, you may be worried about sex positions that involve weight bearing or tenderness around your scar area so try out different positions with your clothes on and see if they feel comfortable.

If sleepless nights and leaking breasts have left you with no sex drive whatsoever, don't panic. Just as you can go off sex, so can partners; they can be exhausted too or put off by watching you go through a difficult birth. Talk to each other, acknowledge the huge change you're both going through and, temporarily, take the pressure off having

sex. Instead, focus on being thoughtful and affectionate. Have a bath together, cuddle as often as you can, and hold hands in bed. Keeping communication open and being tactile means that in time the sex will come.

Remember the sex you have initially may not be the sex you used to have because you may not have the time or energy for it; it's more likely to be something that gives you both release, such as a quickie on the sofa with your clothes on while the baby's having a nap, or even giving each other a massage for five minutes in bed. Think about grabbing snippets of time to be intimate, adding an element of creativity and fun.

If you feel insecure about your new shape, just think about what might help you feel more sexual. It might be having sex under the covers, partially clothed, in the dark or with soft lighting; do what makes you happy for now.

The truth about post-baby contraception: Your OB/GYN may ask you about contraception at some point after the birth, and you should start thinking about it, because you could be just as fertile after having a baby as you were before. You can even become pregnant before your period returns because ovulation occurs about two weeks before you get your period. If you're thinking of having another baby in the next year or so, short-term contraception is best. There are various options for you:

● If you prefer the pill and if you're breastfeeding, a progestogen-only pill is recommended because estrogen may reduce milk flow. This pill can be started immediately after the birth and you take it every day continuously. You won't see any regular bleeding, but some erratic bleeding may occur.

- The combined pill, contraceptive patches or vaginal ring are sometimes recommended if you're not breastfeeding.
- There are many fit-and-forget options if you're too busy (or forgetful) to think about daily contraception. Progestogen-only contraceptive injections can last about twelve weeks, and implants in the arm last for three years. You can have the intrauterine device (IUD), which is inserted vaginally. The hormone-containing type lasts up to five years. A non-hormonal IUD, which releases copper to interfere with sperm, lasts up to ten years. If you want to try for another baby, both can be removed and your fertility will quickly return to normal (it's instant after the IUD is removed). The progestogen-only injection takes longer to wear off, so isn't a good option if you want to get pregnant sooner.
- If you've had a slip-up, the emergency morning-after pill is progestogen-only and can be bought over the counter.
- Then of course, there are condoms, or a cervical cap, which will need resizing post-baby as your cervix and vagina change shape.

REAL LIFE

"I forgot what it was like to want sex"

"For the first four months of Ewan's life, I breastfed constantly and was barely apart from him. I didn't even notice I was totally ignoring my husband. After around ten weeks, my C-section scar was less tender and we tried to have sex, but I wasn't emotionally ready and it felt strange when I was breastfeeding. Joe understood that motherhood had taken over for a while, but I also realized I needed to make an effort so we decided to take it slowly. We started kissing more, and went on date nights and soon I began to fancy him again. Eventually our sex life became something we both wanted to revive, and I'm so glad we took steps to bring the spark back."
STELLA, MOM TO EWAN,
8 MONTHS

YOUR BABY IS GROWING MORE
INTERESTED IN CONVERSATION

....

UNDERSTANDING IMMUNIZATION

....

LEARNING THROUGH PLAY

....

CHAPTER FIVE
BY TWO MONTHS

....

Now that she's two months old, your baby may be
able to hold her head up for a few seconds and follow
objects with her eyes. She'll be strengthening all her
muscles and will become more interested in games.

MAKING CONVERSATION

You'll notice that your baby is becoming more vocal, as the screams and gurgles give way to bird-like "coo" sounds. This is a key milestone in speech development. It's a sign that the muscles of your baby's tongue and mouth are getting stronger and that she is beginning to understand the link between making sounds and getting a reaction from you. So, mirror her sounds. Your baby loves the sound of your voice, so talk, sing, and coo back to her, making as much eye contact as possible. Your child is never too young to make conversation. When she lets out a "coo," repeat it back to her, and she may do the same again. This also teaches her about taking turns—a key skill in conversation.

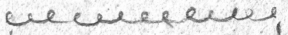

EXPERT TIP

LEARNING LANGUAGE

Research at the University of Washington, suggests that a baby's brain starts laying down the groundwork of how to form words long before they actually begin to speak. Moms seem to know this instinctively as the slow, exaggerated, and high-pitched way they speak to babies—called "mothereze" by experts—makes listening to the mother tongue easier and is key to your baby's learning process. This tone of voice is not just a sign of affection; you're helping your baby learn to distinguish vocal sounds from other noises, which ultimately helps her learn to talk.

DR REBECCA CHICOT
Child development and parenting expert

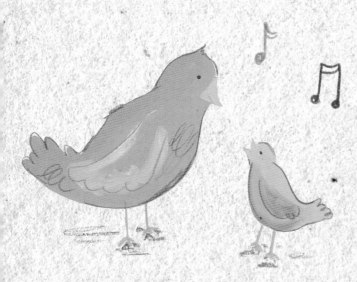

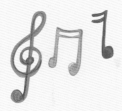

REAL LIFE SLEEP SECRETS

"Bedtime singsong"

"I always sang 'You are my Sunshine' to Joe. After I put him down, I'd hum it by the cot and continue until I made my escape. He was sleeping through at 18 weeks and, if he ever woke, I'd do the same and he'd instantly settle."

SARAH, MOM TO JOE, 19 MONTHS

OUT AND ABOUT WITH A CRYING BABY

Hearing your baby cry is always stressful, but never more so than when you're out in a public place; it can feel that your skills as a mother are suddenly under question. Whether you're out for lunch or at the supermarket, you'll need a few tricks up your sleeve for baby meltdowns.

Check that there's nothing obviously wrong
Try to stay calm and work through a mental checklist of what could be up. Is your baby hungry, tired, or does her diaper need changing? Does she feel hot or seem off color? If you can't find a reason, she may just be having a cranky moment (we all have them), so don't think you are a bad mom.

Pick her up
If you're rushing through the supermarket when your baby wails your stress levels can go through the roof and sometimes it's just not worth soldiering on. Take a pause, pick your baby up, and try to settle her; this may work straight away. If there's no time pressure, you could even head to the supermarket café for a play or a feed.

Change her position
Most young babies actually have certain positions that calms them. The trick is to find them. For a colicky baby, it's often holding her so that her stomach lies flat along your arm, which puts pressure on a sore tummy.

Try a pacifier
If you're someone who can't stand the idea of your baby crying on the bus or in a crowded place, you might want to try a pacifier. It won't prevent crying completely, but it can soothe a baby who's finding it hard to drop off to sleep or is a bit cranky.

UNDERSTANDING IMMUNIZATION

Your baby is born with little immune defence against the world around her. She needs to develop her own resistance and will have help in the form of the baby immunization program which starts at birth in the US. Immunizations prevent serious and potentially fatal diseases such as meningitis. They are mostly delivered as injections and will help your baby's immune system fight off potentially serious diseases, from rotavirus, a common gastric bug, to diphtheria, measles, hemophilus influenza type b (a bacterial infection that can lead to meningitis), and pneumonia, which can lead to another form of meningitis. Some immunizations are combined into one injection and your baby's pediatrician will give her a series of injections at different stages. As more and more research is developed the list of potential immunizations changes. Talk to the pediatrician about the latest recommendations and timings.

The pediatrician's office should let you know when your baby is due for each vaccine, but if you think you've been forgotten then do follow it up. Your baby will also have a full health check at two months.

Keeping your baby calm

While the injections may not be pleasant for her at the time, the benefits far out way the discomfort. There are ways to help her. Your biggest goal is to keep her still!

Use whatever method or game your baby usually loves to take her attention away from the big needle heading towards her. Take your baby's favorite toy to play with, pull silly faces, sing that embarrassing song she loves or look through a picture book together.

If you're breastfeeding, try feeding her while the injection is given. It involves skin-to-skin contact and lots of love—which your baby can never get enough of. Breastmilk is also full of endorphins, the hormones that naturally suppress pain. If you don't breastfeed, giving her a pacifier to suck on can be a great problem solver.

Our skin is more sensitive when we're cold, so keep her warm when she's having an injection. Babies love, and crave, reassurance; your little baby wants you to cuddle and kiss her and tell her she's OK once the injection is over and done with.

Finally, rubbing your baby's skin gently, close to where she was injected, for about ten seconds, will help. The sensation will distract from the sting of the injection and may help your baby feel the pain less.

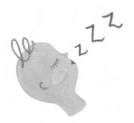

REAL LIFE SLEEP SECRETS

....

"Calming tricks"

"Jack used to scream at bedtime, which made me feel helpless. Then I read how stroking a child's nose in a downward motion can be soothing and encourage them to close their eyes; I tried it successfully. Now, even if I have to go to him in the night, it takes less than five minutes to get him back to sleep."

SHELLEY, MOM TO JACK, 21 MONTHS

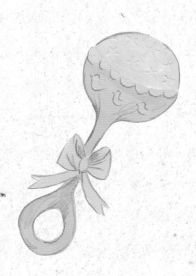

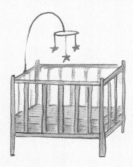

REAL LIFE SLEEP SECRETS

"Limit distractions"

"We used to have mobiles, loads of toys, and glowing stars in Sophie's room, but she still screamed at bedtime and when she woke in the night. My friend pointed out how busy her nursery was, so we removed most of the gadgets and she slept better."

ELLIE, MOM TO SOPHIE, TEN MONTHS

DID YOU KNOW?

The combination of seeing an object and hearing sound also teaches your baby cause and effect.

LEARNING THROUGH PLAY

Seeing your baby master a new skill—and be suitably proud of herself—is a very exciting moment for every parent. Of course, the trick is to make learning seem like one great big game. Become your baby's favorite playmate. The most important games are basic, everyday ones that allow you to share a moment of joy, discovery, or connection. For example, crouching beside your baby on a play mat and shaking a rattle can encourage her to turn her head and she may even roll over for the first time. In those first months, get your baby grabbing for toys in her baby bouncer or swing by holding them just a little out of reach.

Try "throw and float"
Lay your baby on her back, crumple some brightly colored fabric into a ball, throw it into the air, and let it float down onto her. This helps your baby's visual tracking. Tell your baby what you are doing, too, that way she's also using her hearing, seeing, and touching senses.

Play "peek-a-boo"
This is a great game for all babies of any age—her laughter will make you feel like a comic genius. Hide your face, wait for a few seconds, then reappear saying, "peek-a-boo!" This game helps your baby understand

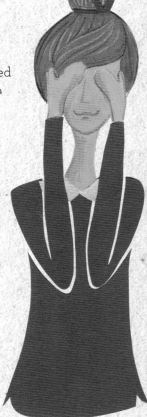

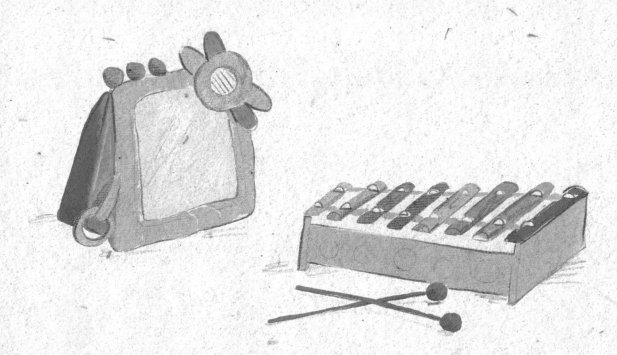

that when something (or someone) isn't visible, it still exists—a concept called object permanence. Children don't fully grasp this concept until they're at least 18 months old; at this stage it simply helps your baby understand that although you might disappear, you'll come back. Waiting for you to "reappear" develops her attention and concentration skills.

The mirror game
This is a great game for tummy time. Put a play mirror on the floor and lie on your tummy beside your baby. Stick your tongue out and make faces in the mirror so your baby can see you. Not all babies enjoy "tummy time," so playing with a mirror can distract her from the fact she's on her front. This game is great when your baby is strong enough to lift her head and shoulders up when lying on her tummy—usually around three months.

Make music together
Shake an instrument or play some music and clap your hands in time to it. Eventually your baby will be old enough to play with the instrument herself. As well as setting your baby on the road to being a music virtuoso, there are plenty of other benefits to this game, for example, learning to find a rhythm is great for language development and even math.

Making more mom friends

Adjusting to a new life with your baby can be made easier if you know other people in the same position. Who else is going to understand why you're awake in the early hours (and know what it feels like), or that you are beyond excited that your local cinema has started doing mom-and-baby screenings? Take advantage of the other opportunities for expanding your local social circle and finding like-minded moms to arrange coffee or play dates with. They give you a chance to have a catch up with a fellow mom while your tots take in the world. You'll be glad you did.

Get chatty

Be confident to strike up a conversation with other moms and be open about your experiences of motherhood—it will make other moms feel comfortable opening up to you. Who knows, the local supermarket baby supplies aisle could be your new socializing hub.

Join baby groups

Get out and about with your baby by attending weekly baby groups. Lots of libraries hold weekly storytelling sessions for moms and kids. Swimming or baby yoga classes can be great places to amuse you and your baby and they're a source of other parents. Ask your pediatrician about groups in your area.

Make the most of support groups

You can make friends at support groups too. For example, don't be afraid to talk about something other than latching on and nipples at your breastfeeding group.

Multi-task when you're exercising

The gym, exercise classes, and stroller fit groups in the park are all great places to get chatting to other moms, especially if there's a crèche. You could even suggest meeting for coffee and cake as a pat on the back for all your fitness efforts.

Embrace waiting rooms

Your pediatrician's office waiting room—or anywhere you sit around with other parents—can be good place to strike up a conversation. Obviously gauge the situation and choose people who actually look like they want to be spoken to. It doesn't hurt to try to chat while you wait as your babies give you common ground, especially if they look like they are a similar age.

Make a date with a friend

Meet up with a friend for coffee and suggest each of you brings someone else the other doesn't know. It makes a first meeting way less awkward.

Stay connected

If none of your friends have had babies yet, meeting up with some of the women from your antenatal classes is the ideal way to bring some mom friends into your life. You'll be able to compare what you're going through and indulge in a gossip.

Hit social media

Twitter's an open community and loads of parents make some of their closest friends through it. Follow *Mother&Baby* on Facebook and Twitter, and check out our hashtag "#nightfeed" when you're awake at two o'clock in the morning.

When everyone else is sleeping, it is comforting to know there are other moms out there going through the same thing as you.

Check out the internet

What's helpful is that pretty much all parents acknowledge they're in the same social boat and enjoy talking to others in the same situation. Many of the parenting websites have sections dedicated to connecting people locally.

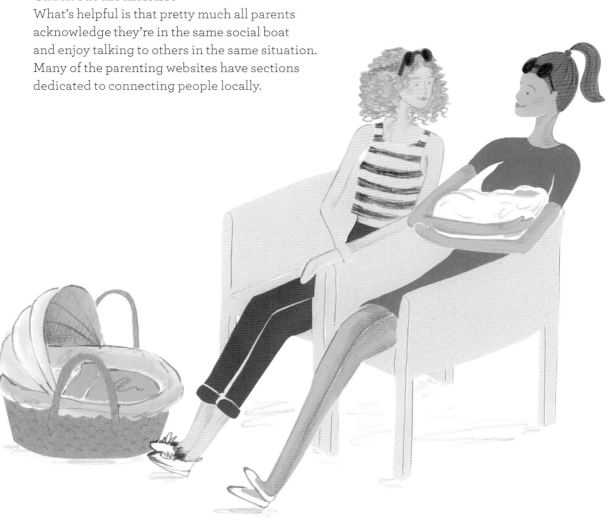

CHAPTER SIX
FROM THREE MONTHS

You baby will probably be getting five good milk feeds now, from his first morning feed to his late evening feed. He will probably wake for a feed in the night. He should be having between three and three quarter hours and four and a quarter hours of daytime sleep.

YOUR BABY IS DEVELOPING FAST

By the time your baby is three months old, he'll have developed some appreciation of you as a person. He'll recognize that you're his mom and enjoy being talked to and looked at by his parents and close family. He'll also have better head control and will start to gently kick, wriggle, and may even be able to roll from his back on to his stomach or vice versa. His hand-to-eye coordination is getting better and he may try to bat rattles or hanging toys away. As your baby's muscles develop, he will start to reach out for and grasp things too. Ensure you have interesting playthings for him to explore; look for colorful toys that make sounds to spark his curiosity.

Your baby will also start putting things in his mouth. Researchers from the Institute of Cognitive Sciences, France, believe this is down to a survival instinct. It is also a way of examining objects. His brain is learning about different textures and it's easier to put objects in his mouth than to examine them with his hands and eyes. Just ensure there are no choking hazards around and watch him to make sure he stays safe.

Talk to your baby all the time

Now is a great time to interact verbally with your baby; tell him what you're doing and why. For example, if you're in the kitchen making breakfast, explain what you're doing. Even though he still seems so young, this helps him learn about language and conversational skills.

EXPERT TIP

WORRIED ABOUT DEVELOPMENT?

While it's important to relax and remember that all babies develop at different rates, it's essential to speak to your baby's pediatrician if you have any concerns about your child's development, for example if he's not smiling by the age of three months, or if he's slow to develop several skills. Above all, trust your instincts as a mother and never be afraid to raise any concerns you have.

DR REBECCA CHICOT
Child development and parenting expert

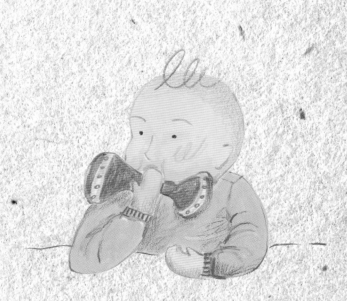

BABY CLASSES

There are lots classes available for babies from birth to six months, which are not only brilliant for getting you out and about, but also really help the bond between you and your baby develop. Your pediatrician may be able to direct you to some. Going to classes when your baby is this age is about stimulating his senses through movement, music or simply new experiences. But it's not all about your baby. These classes provide another opportunity to meet other moms going through the same life stage. So go with a view to bonding with your baby and making some new friends.

Postnatal groups are a useful place to get answers to your babycare questions or to learn new techniques such as baby massage. Ask your pediatrician about groups in your area. Some of the options available are opposite.

Baby swimming classes
A time to have fun in the water with your baby as well as give him a head start when it comes to swimming. Get online to find groups where you live, or see Resources (page 155) for some ideas.

Sensory baby classes
These are great for introducing your baby to new sights, sounds, and sensations. The classes are varied and fun and include music, singing, bubbles, and other experiences to help your baby try new things.

Baby massage classes
Massage is a great way to bond with your baby. You can also learn techniques that help ease colic and help you both get a good night's sleep. Search the internet for baby massage classes in your area or ask your pediatrician.

Baby yoga classes
These classes usually combine traditional yoga techniques with movements, gentle stretches and calm breathing techniques.

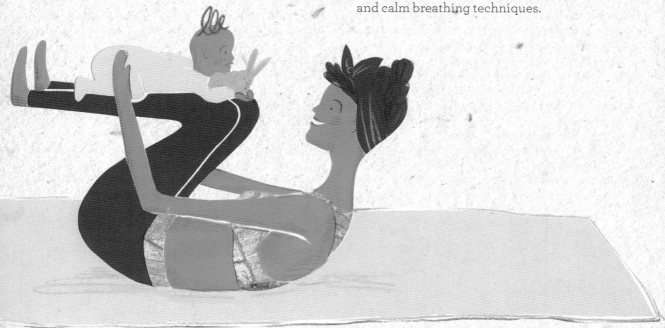

BABY PERSONALITIES

Your baby is one in a million. Whether it's his fits of giggles at your silly voice or his ability to take just about everything in his stride, your baby's personality is unique to him.

Birth order

Your baby's place in the family affects his attitude to success. Research has shown that firstborns tend to judge their achievements by how they stack up against their own past abilities, while second siblings tend to compare themselves to others. Your youngest child could be the most creative. He's the baby, so he's put in that center-of-attention role. As a parent, you may also be more relaxed through experience, so your youngest toddler can take more risks, which naturally leads to discovery and creativity.

Feeding style can affect personality

Is your breastfed baby headstrong? It is often the case, according to research by the Medical Research Council in Cambridge, UK. In a study of 316 three-month-old babies, the breastfed infants took longer to calm down after excitement compared with those who were bottle-fed.

Avoid stereotypes

Reconsider before choosing a blue blanket for a boy—according to a study, all babies are drawn to reds over blues. And who needs gender stereotypes? If he sees you driving and his dad cooking—and vice versa—he won't feel restricted by basic ideas of what men and women do.

Social life

Temperament is something your baby is born with, but it's the experiences he has that will

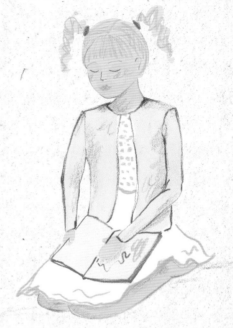

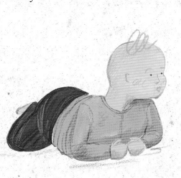

work with his natural temperament to form his personality. If he's sensitive, new situations like mom-and-toddler groups may make him anxious, so introduce him gradually. You can boost your baby's social skills by letting him be around other children. Babies are fascinated by each other and interaction helps their confidence build and develop.

Being silly

Want your baby to have a good sense of humor? When it comes to what we find funny, humor is pretty innate and very personal, but you can help your toddler to express his funny side regularly by playing, singing, and laughing with him.

Expose him to adult conversation

Rather than sticking to baby talk, try upping your grown-up chat around your child. Only children are often more confident from an early age and tend to be very verbal because they're mainly surrounded by adult conversation. Talk to your friends and older children in front of your baby or toddler—you'll be amazed at how much he absorbs.

CHOOSING CHILDCARE

You might be going back to work around now, or just looking at your options. It is a good idea to look at these well in advance. Your instincts will often tell you whether an individual or nursery is right for your child, but asking the right questions can help you make an informed choice.

What are the choices?

When it comes to childcare, there are various factors to consider: if you choose a daycare center or in-home daycare your child will be away from home; if you opt for a nanny and possibly au pair she can be based at home. Daycare centers try to consider your personal preferences but, generally, your child will fit in with the established routine, whereas in-home daycarers and nannies can be more parent-led. Make a list of the pros and cons for each type. You'll also need to consider your work commitments—nannies and aupairs will likely be more flexible if you need irregular hours. Cost is another vital factor too. Some employers offer a Flexible Spending Account, allowing you pre-tax dollars for eligible childcare expenses. Ask your human resources department what they do.

There are more flexible types of childcare springing up too. Pop-up crèches are popular at co-working spaces (hubs for freelancers or people who run their own business to rent desk space),

and wraparound childcare is another new trend, which is when someone comes to your house to cover late shifts, early drop offs, and holiday and weekend care. Ask friends and other moms about local options.

You can find may find individuals' reviews for daycare centers, but you'll also learn a lot from visiting and watching other children there. As well as seeing how happy they seem, talk to the staff and other parents. Ask what they enjoy about working there, or what their favorite activity is for the children. If you don't like what you see, move on. You probably made the decision about where to live based on instinct, and you should listen to this when it comes to childcare. Most moms will get a good feeling about the place they choose. Ask yourself, "Can I imagine my child here? Will they be happy? Will their care and welfare needs be met?"

Before you go back to work

If you've barely spent time away from your baby until now, it's a good idea to get him used to being looked after by other people. Leave him with a close friend or relatives while you go out for a few hours. This will introduce the idea that sometimes mommy goes away, but that she always comes back.

Try not to show any anxiety about your return to work. Even if you think you're just chatting about it with a mom friend, children are experts at picking up on your feelings. If they are a little bit older, make sure you're positive about childcare whenever you discuss it in front of your little one.

Preparing your child for daycare

When you have decided to go back to work, prepare your child as well as yourself. Tell stories about children going to daycare—talking to your little one in a relaxed way about his new routine and reading children's books about going to daycare, or mommy going to work, can really help.

DID YOU KNOW?

You may also be able to take part in nanny share, splitting the hours or services of a nanny with one other family.

QUESTIONS FOR A DAYCARE CENTER OR IN-HOME DAYCARE

"What qualifications do you/the staff have?"

Qualifications in childcare prove that a daycare worker or nanny has a good understanding of your baby's needs and how he'll develop. Ideally, daycare center staff should have a recognized childcare qualification. Someone who runs an in-home daycare is less likely to have qualifications, but it's a good idea to check she holds a license, CPR, and first-aid certificate.

"Will my baby be safe?"

Do a bit of digging and find official reports about the nursery to highlight any problems with safety and welfare. You want to feel that a carer is on the ball; you can glean a lot from watching childcare in action, so look out for children being left with runny noses, crying without being comforted, or drifting about unsupervised.

"What will the daily routine be?"

If you employ a nanny, your baby's existing routine should stay pretty much the same. This may be true for an in-home daycare depending on how many children she is looking after. At a daycare center, he may be encouraged to fit in with the others, taking one big nap after dinner, for example, but staff should offer to be flexible while your baby adapts to daycare center life.

"How will I be kept informed of progress?"

Daycare workers should keep a developmental record of your baby, which should be sent home every so often; feel free to add comments of your own. Your baby will also have a key worker at a daycare center for you to talk to about concerns. With a nanny or au pair, it's helpful for her to write down what your child's done each day, including what he's eaten, and when he slept.

"What about discipline?"

Of course, a baby would never be considered naughty at this age. However, general boundaries are essential to keep your baby safe and happy. Some daycare centers are stricter than others, but the exact approach should be set out in its policy documents, which you can ask to see. When you visit a daycare center or in-home daycare, keep an eye out for behavioral incidents to see how they're handled. Ideally, the careworker should deal with situations on the spot, then move on.

If you're going for a daycare center, try to approach a few of the other parents about setting up a playdate with some other children who will be in the same group. If your baby hasn't been in a social setting before, this is a great idea as it will be a big change to spend time in the company of other kids. And you might even score yourself some new mommy mates, too.

Just as it will take time for you to settle back into work (goodbye coffee shop, hello office), it's the same for your child, so ease him into nursery gently. Begin with an hour there together, then a couple of hours without you, finally building up to a full day. And tempting as it may be to sneak out while your baby is assessing the toy selection, he can panic when he realizes you're not there. Even if it makes him cry, tell your child you're leaving and that you'll see him again soon. Then give him a time-related reference, like "Mommy will be back at teatime." Leave him with a comforter to remind him of home, such as a blanket, favorite cuddly toy or pacifier. Leave something of yours too, such as a scarf, and ask him to look after it until you return, reinforcing the idea that you're coming back. Once you've decided to go, do it. Lingering will let him know you're anxious.

QUESTIONS FOR A NANNY

Think about asking the following:

- ○ How much childcare experience do you have?
- ○ Do you have qualifications and/or a first aid certificate?
- ○ Can you provide at least two written references (and their phone numbers)?
- ○ What are your salary expectations?
- ○ What hours are you willing to work?
- ○ Are you willing to work occasional weekends and sit on occasion?
- ○ Are you willing to do household chores?
- ○ What did you like most/least about your last job?
- ○ If offered the job, how long do you intend to work here?
- ○ How do you encourage good behavior in children?

Following up the interview

Try to speak to the referees on the phone—a chat can reveal more than a written reference. Ask to see certificates for qualifications; if they've been lost, phone up the college to confirm the course was completed. Once you have a shortlist, arrange for a prospective nanny or au pair to spend some time with your child to see how they get on.

Choosing a nanny

A nanny can be a great option if you would prefer for your child to be looked after in your own home, need daycare outside of normal working hours or have more than one pre-school child. Nannies often have childcare qualifications. Some families find that a live-in nanny works best for them, while others choose to hire on a day basis.

If you employ a live-in nanny, you will need to provide her with meals and her own bedroom in addition to a salary. Many families also provide a car or pay petrol expenses if the nanny has her own vehicle. Day nannies come into the home each day and work a set number of hours (generally a maximom of 10 a day) and go home in the evening.

What is an au pair?

Au pairs tend to be young, single people who work alongside you in the home and may complete chores as well as help take care of the children. They are rarely trained to work with children, so are usually unlikely to be suitable for looking after babies or pre-school children while you're out at work. Many au pairs come from overseas, and choose to live with a family while they are studying the language. They can only work a certain number of hours and must have at one or two full days off each week. You will need to provide an au pair with his or her own bedroom, meals, and an allowance.

Employing a nanny

As your nanny's employer, it's your responsibility to sort out salary and any extras such as tax so take this into account when working out costs. Once your chosen candidate has accepted the job, you'll need to draw up a contract. This should outline your expectations (along with what happens with sick leave and holidays) and should help prevent problems occurring further down the line. Be sure to include daily duties and hours of work: will you want your nanny to sit one Saturday in the month? Do you require him or her to be flexible if you're going away for a business trip? Also state whether you intend for there to be a probationary period and a procedure for terminating the contract— for example a month's notice on either side.

DEALING WITH COLDS

If your baby is snuffly, he might well have a cold; babies and toddlers have them all the time. Typical symptoms include a blocked or runny nose, a raised temperature (over 99.5°F), cough, loss of appetite, and irritability. Monitor his temperature and if it is high remove some of his clothes and give plenty of fluids. If he is distressed you can also give medication to bring down his temperature such as infant acetaminophen. Check wi your doctor before giving ibuprofen top a baby under six months. Always follow the directions on the packet and never exceed the stated dose. Don't medicate a baby under three months unless advised to by your doctor. Contact your baby's pediatrician if you are concerned and definitely seek medical advice straight away if your child is floppy or drowsy.

Treating a blocked nose

If your baby's nose is blocked, he may struggle to breathe through it, so feeding can be difficult. A baby saline nasal spray or drops can help loosen trapped mucus. You can then use a nasal aspirator to gently and safely suction out any nasal congestion. Putting a humidifier in the room can also help to ease congestion.

Can a cold be prevented?

Although you can't really prevent a cold, sensible hygiene measures, such as keeping your baby away from anyone who has one, and disinfecting surfaces that have been sneezed on, can help to keep your child healthy and feeling well.

Staying well hydrated will also give your child's own immune system the ability to recover more quickly from a cold, should he pick any more up.

EXPERT TIP

COULD IT BE A CHEST INFECTION?

Most infections in the chest are due to viruses and can be bronchiolitis, bronchitis, or pneumonia. They are worse than a heavy cold and bronchiolitis is extremely common, affecting about a third of babies in their first year. Speak to your doctor if you think your baby has a chest infection.

Preemies or those born with severe heart or lung problems are more likely to contract chest infections. The more severe chest infections are usually bacterial, spurred on by an original viral illness. Make sure your baby is up to date with routine immunisations, which will help to prevent infections such as whooping cough (pertussis).

There are symptoms that indicate a chest infection. Coughing and fast breathing are the most common, but an infant can also have irregular breathing or pauses in breathing without a fever. The infection itself may last just five to seven days, but the symptoms can last much longer.

DR PHILIPPA KAYE
Family doctor

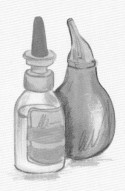

REAL LIFE

"A runny nose and cough were the first signs of his cold"

"I first noticed Reuben had a runny nose and it sounded like he had a sore throat. He was coughing, too, but he didn't have a temperature. This was his first cold, but I guessed there was something wrong because of his symptoms and the fact that he was quite grumpy—he's usually a very happy baby. He was also waking more often in the night and feeding less but more often. I got a saline spray, which helped clear his nose. The cold lasted three days before it got better— and none of us got much sleep that week."

JENNY, MOM TO REUBEN, 15 WEEKS

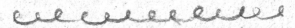

EXPERT TIP

WHEN HE IS UNWELL

You may find that feeding your baby is difficult as he has to suck, breathe, and swallow all at the same time—tricky when he is already finding it harder to breathe than normal. Chest infections leave infants younger than three months old exhausted as they have to breathe through their nose. Your baby may wheeze due to the narrowing or secretions in the lower airways.

DR PHILIPPA KAYE
Family doctor

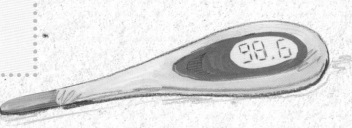

····· How to feel healthier and more energized ·····

Yes, it is possible to feel really good after having a baby!

Drink up

Our bodies are made up of 65 per cent water; it's needed for everything from bodily functions to concentration. Drinking water may help to support the immune system, soothe sore throats, and replenish fluids lost through sneezing and forming mucus when you have a cold (and through breastfeeding).

Strengthen your immunity

As colds are spread through coughing, sneezing, and contact with contaminated surfaces, use a hand sanitizer. Keep an eye on your sugar intake; too much can suppress your immune system. Include a wide range of brightly colored fruit and vegetables in your diet to boost your antioxidants. If you have a fever, don't press on; call back-up childcare and go to bed.

Boost your mood with light

Light is important for your mood, alertness, and sleep patterns. In the winter months, many people feel low and can struggle to get up in the mornings—it's known as seasonal affective disorder (SAD). Ease symptoms by spending at least an hour out of doors in the middle of the day, or by using a light box that replicates sunshine. You can buy lamps that incorporate a simulated sunrise and sunset alarm clock and emit a calming aromatherapy spray.

Tactics to increase energy

You'll have your best-quality sleep between 10.30pm and 1.30am, so try to make sure you are in bed at that time. If you wake up feeling tired, try side stretches to lengthen muscles and help you take deeper, more energizing breaths. Stand with your feet hip-distance apart and sweep the arms up over the head, interlacing the fingers and rolling the palms up. Inhale as you straighten up, and exhale as you side bend over to your right; repeat to the left.

How to feel refreshed

Nights out may seem like a distant memory, but if you're having the odd glass of wine try ginger tea to calm the stomach (ask your pediatrician about safe alcohol consumption while you are breastfeeding). Top up your levels of vitamin B and C, either with a supplement or eat plenty of fresh fruit and vegetables; vitamin C protects the liver, while vitamin B gives an energy boost. A cooling shower with a refreshing citrus shower gel can help to wake you up for the day ahead too.

NOTES

NEWBORN TO 3 MONTHS

NEWBORN

Try to make sure you have all your newborn essentials ready for a couple of weeks before your due date, there'll be lots more to think about when your baby arrives!

Have you been trying tummy time? Just make sure you stay with him the whole time.

WEEK 3

Your baby will need to feed regularly, every two to three hours, as his tummy is so tiny.

WEEK 1

Don't worry about creating a strict routine for now and focus on establishing eating habits, keeping him warm and cuddled with lots of consistent care from you and your partner so he feels safe and secure.

NEWBORN

NEWBORN

When your baby arrives there'll be lots of opportunities for you and your partner to bond with him, but try to have as much skin-on-skin time together as possible straight after the birth.

Your baby's first poo will be formed from meconium, a dark, green-black sticky substance but will soften in a few days to yellow poos to reflect his new milk diet.

There are lots of firsts to learn about at this stage including your baby's first bath, getting to grips with feeding, whether you decide to bottle or breast feed, and starting to recognize your baby's different cries and what they signify.

It's time for your post-natal check-up—the 6 week check for you.

WEEK 6

WEEK 6

At any point from one to three months old your baby will start to lift his head.

Your baby will to smile on his own around now—any time from six to 12 weeks.

MONTH 2

Your baby is becoming more vocal, and making cooing and gurgling sounds.

MONTH 3

He'll also start exploring more and will put things into his mouth as a way to do this.

Talk to him lots and try out new baby classes to interact with other babies, moms, and dads.

MONTH 3

Your baby may even be able to roll now—never put him on a raised surface and leave him unattended.

He has better head control and will start kicking and moving more as well as showing better hand-to-eye coordination.

If you have decided to go back to work, this is probably the time when you will be leaving your baby in the care of the daycare center, in-home daycare, nanny, or au pair that you've chosen.

MONTH 3

Now is the time to try out lots of games to help with aspects of your baby's development including visual tracking, learning object permanence, developing attention, and concentration.

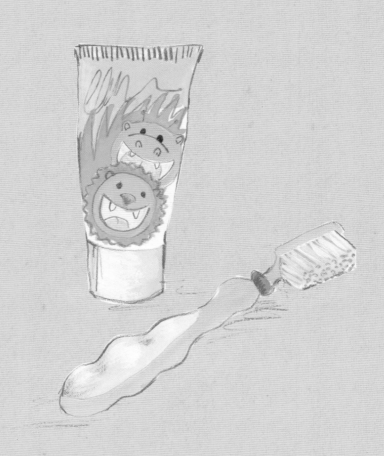

FOUR TO SEVEN MONTHS

CHAPTER SEVEN
FROM FOUR MONTHS

You'll be continuing with five good milk feeds a day. But the difference now is that if your baby is over 14lbs, she should be able to sleep through without a night feed. During the day your baby should nap for around four hours in total.

SHE'S REALLY COMMUNICATING NOW

Your baby will begin to make different noises around now and may be babbling, although she won't start imitating speech sounds until she's six months. At this stage she will start to realize that if she makes a noise she'll get a reaction, so try sticking out your tongue and letting your baby copy what you do. She's learning to take turns, which is a version of pre-verbal speech.

Your baby's hand-eye coordination will be developing fast. She's learning to give and take objects and will be able to hold a comforter or soft rattle. She'll also track objects and people with her eyes now. She should have fairly good head control by now, and may be able to roll over (although this may not happen until seven months), and lift her head and shoulders off the floor when she's lying on her tummy or back.

EXPERT TIP

ENCOURAGING YOUR BABY'S MOBILITY

Your baby's motor skills are gearing up at this age. Babies start to realize that they can grab things and move them from one hand to the other. Whereas a newborn baby instinctively grasps her mother's finger, by four months your baby is consciously grabbing things. Give your baby lots of clean and safe things to play with and explore to help develop her motor skills. She loves things like books (choose cardboard ones for now), toys, spoons, and objects with lots of different colors and textures.

If she's slow to roll, give her more "tummy time." It's been found that because young babies are put down to sleep on their backs (to reduce the risk of cot death), motor skills like rolling may be slightly delayed. Counter this by ensuring plenty of tummy time during the day.

PENNY LAZELL
Healthcare professional

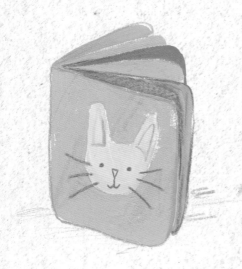

EXPERT TIP

BABY SLEEP

One thing that will make your day much easier is a structure. This means choosing a time that suits you as a "getting-up" time (it needs to be consistent, so pick one that you're happy with) and a "bedtime." You can then plan when your baby is going to need her naps. Between waking up and bedtime (roughly 12 hours) she needs to have around four hours sleep. This structure can be the basis for the routine that will help settle your baby.

Most moms have a start time that coincides with when their baby tends to wake up, but if you need to start your day earlier, you'll need to gently rouse your little one. Removing a sleep sack will change her temperature, which often prompts her to stir. You can also open the curtains to let in some natural light. Let your baby come round in her own way, and speak to her gently, so she knows you're there.

TINA SOUTHWOOD
Sleep consultant

Q&A

"What happens if she rolls over at night?"

Sleep consultant **TINA SOUTHWOOD** says, "Once your baby starts rolling you may have a period where you have a few broken nights when she rolls in her sleep. When babies roll and bump themselves, or get their arms stuck through the bars of their crib, it can wake them. Many parents worry about their baby rolling onto her tummy in the night. If you see she's done it, roll her back onto her back again, but remember that she may turn herself straight back onto her tummy. You cannot stay up all night watching to make sure that your baby doesn't roll; your baby has now got strong muscles in her head and her back and she can lift her head off the mattress. If you need to feel more reassured about this, just give her plenty of tummy time during the day. That way you she can build her strength and you can see her practising her rolling."

TEETHING BEGINS

Your baby's primary, or milk, teeth begin to cut through the gums soon. This can happen somewhere between six and nine months of age, but it can happen a lot earlier. Rarely, a baby has a tooth present at birth, but all of her milk teeth will have come through by the time she is three years old.

Some babies sail through teething with no problem at all, whereas others seem to become extremely irritable, cry a lot, become clingy and/ or don't sleep well. Teething babies may dribble more, which can result in a slight rash around the mouth. Your baby might try to thrust her fist into her mouth in an attempt to chew it. Other signs of teething include going off food because her mouth is painful and she may pull at her ears. You might notice a lump on the gum, which looks red and swollen; as the tooth breaks through you may feel a hard lump with your fingertip. A few months later when the larger back teeth come through, your child's cheek can look red and feel hot to the touch.

Some doctors and dentists dismiss the idea that teething can cause other generalized symptoms, but others are convinced that they can. Some believe symptoms including earache, a slight temperature or vomiting and diarrhoea can coincide with teething, but always see your baby's pediatrician if your baby seems unwell.

How you can help

It's well worth buying some of the products designed to ease the pain of teething. Soothe gums with teething gels, which are available over the counter. Some contain a local anesthetic—usually lidocaine—that numbs the soreness and an antiseptic to prevent infections. Your baby will naturally chew on things now, so give her a teething toy; they're made of special materials

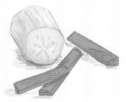

REAL LIFE

"Teething products worked for my daughter"

"Charlotte started teething at 20 weeks old. I noticed her cheeks looked flushed and she was crying more. I used teething gels and dampened her favorite comforter with iced water and she'd happily chew on that. Once we started solids after six months and she was eating baby food, she would often have days where she'd be off her food. When I fed her warm purées, I'd put a dollop of yoghurt on top, which helped cool them down."
ALISON, MOM TO CHARLOTTE, NINE MONTHS

that won't crack or break when she bites on them. Put them in the fridge for a while before giving them to your baby as the cold can soothe your baby's gums. Likewise, offer her a cold, damp washcloth or burp cloth to chew on; the slightly rough texture massages the gums.

You'll probably find teething doesn't cause as many problems during the day, as your baby is distracted by what's going on around her. However, at night, she may wake up repeatedly. If this is the case, rub a little teething gel on her gums, cuddle her, then gently encourage her back to sleep. You could also give infant acetaminophen if she seems to be in a lot of discomfort (follow the instructions on the pack, always check your baby is old enough and weighs enough to have the medicine and never exceed the stated dose). By and large, it's not a good idea to rely on this too much as teething can go on for quite a long time and too much acetaminophen can be potentially harmful.

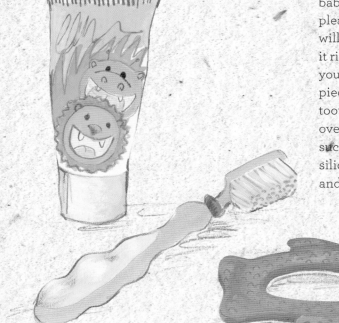

Help her enjoy toothbrush time!

As soon as your baby's teeth start to come through, you can start brushing them. Use a baby toothbrush with a tiny smear of baby toothpaste and make it a fun, relaxed, and pleasant experience for her. Don't worry if you don't manage to brush much at first. To begin with, just let her chew on the brush so she gets used to it. She'll enjoy the feel of the bristles on her gums and this can prevent her becoming reluctant to clean her teeth as she gets older.

The easiest way to brush a baby's teeth is to sit her on your knee with her head resting against your chest. Brush the tooth or teeth using small circular movements, twice a day with a fluoride-free toothpaste developed for your baby's age, so that its formula, mild flavor, and active ingredients will be suitable (adult toothpaste contains too much fluoride and could damage developing teeth).

Be very gentle, there is no need to scrub! Your baby's first experience of tooth care needs to be a pleasant one so, as long as she is comfortable and willing to let you brush her teeth, you are getting it right. If she doesn't like her baby toothbrush, you can clean your baby's teeth by wrapping a piece of damp gauze with a tiny amount of baby toothpaste on it over your finger and rubbing this over her teeth, or there are products on the market such as chewable baby toothbrushes with soft silicone bristles to help to keep both the teeth and gums clean.

Your first night out

You've been looking forward to your first post-baby night out for weeks. You are longing for an undisturbed glass of wine and grown-up conversation, but suddenly you have a bad case of nerves (and you thought separation anxiety only happened to babies). Don't stress, there are ways to stay calm and keep your baby happy.

Whether it's your mom, a friend, or sitter, if you're leaving your baby in the hands of someone else for the first time, knowing that she's in an environment that she knows and recognizes will help put your mind at ease. If you are leaving her with a sitter, talk to other people who have used him or her. Once you hear how good their experience was you will feel so much more relaxed and confident.

Explain your bedtime routine

If you're going out before your baby goes to bed, make sure your care provider knows how you like to run your routine—such as bath, feed, story, bed—then even if it's not you putting your baby down, she'll recognize the sleep cues, and will feel safe. Always make sure whoever is looking after your baby has had time with you and your little one beforehand so he or she can see how you do things. For example, what position does your baby like for her feed, how does she prefer to be burped, what does she have in her cot. All these things will help you and your baby to feel relaxed.

Give your baby a familiar burp cloth or leave one of your T-shirts with your sitter as it will have your unique scent, which your baby will recognize. Then whoever's looking after your baby can let her nuzzle it if she's feeling upset. This classic solution has been used for centuries and it really works. Your baby will feel that her mommy is around and it helps her to relax and sleep.

Your separation anxiety is the other side of the parenting coin

A healthy bond with your child means a certain degree of discomfort when you are not with her. Your goal isn't to get rid of worry or doubt, in fact, nerves are part of our parenting instinct and they help us make good decisions. Remember, you're probably much more stressed than your baby, and this is normal. As long as your baby is fed, kept clean, warm, and loved she will be absolutely fine.

It can be tempting to bombard the babysitter with texts and calls every 20 minutes to find out what's going on at home, but it's worth limiting yourself to one call or text to check your little one is happy and then go and enjoy a drink and the company of your friends and your partner.

CHAPTER EIGHT
FROM FIVE MONTHS

By around five months your baby will begin to lift objects and suck them—this is the start of him putting everything in his mouth, so look for colorful non-toxic toys he can explore. From three months to seven-plus months, and once your baby's neck muscles are strong enough, he'll learn to roll over.

BABY SAFETY

Having a small person in the house opens up the possibility of a range of accidents. It's difficult when you have a baby desperate to explore the world, but you can take steps to prevent accidents. Your baby may not be able to move very far just yet and some of the following advice will be more relevant to older babies, but think about baby-proofing your home sooner rather than later, so you're prepared when he does get going.

Often, children are so absorbed in their own immediate interests they are oblivious to their surroundings. They only have a limited perception of the environment because of their lack of experience or development, so are unaware of the consequences of situations that they encounter. Plus, being small, inquisitive, and with a tendency to show off or over-reach their abilities they're more likely to put themselves at risk.

Reduce the risk of falls

Falls are by far the most common causes of accidents in the home and account for 44 per cent of all children's accidents. Most falls involve tripping over on the same level, but the most serious consequences result from falls between two levels, such as falling out of a stroller or highchair or falling from a bed, or down the stairs. Fit a safety gate at the top and bottom of stairs and repair or replace damaged or worn carpet to avoid tripping hazards. Likewise, don't leave items on the stairs. Don't place furniture under a window as a child could climb up it, and ensure your windows have locks or a safety device.

Preventing burns and scalds

A child's skin is much more sensitive than an adult's and a hot drink can still be warm enough to burn a child 15 minutes after it was made. Never hold a hot drink when you are carrying your child. Always put hot drinks out of reach, well away from the edges of tables and worktops.

When running a bath, turn the cold tap on first, then add the hot water. Always test the water temperature with your elbow before letting a child get in. Keep your child away from the taps. Many scalds happen when a child gets into the bath before it's ready, he plays near the hot tap when he's in the bath or if he leans over the edge to pick out a toy and falls into the hot water.

Children can also suffer burns after contact with open fires, a cooker, irons, curling tongs, and hair straighteners, cigarettes, matches, and cigarette lighters so keep them out of reach of children, even when they're cooling down.

Keep your baby out of the kitchen if possible. Use back burners on the stove when possible and turn the panhandles away from the front of the stove so your child won't be able to grab them.

Be careful with glass

Contact with glass can cause severe bleeding. When buying furniture that incorporates glass, look for safety standard marks, which show that it's specially reinforced. If you break a glass always clear it quickly, make sure there are no tiny shards on the floor. Dispose of it safely by wrapping it in newspaper before placing it in the bin.

TAKE ACTION

If your child is injured and bleeding, has a burn, breathing difficulties, or has swallowed something dangerous, take him straight to your local emergency room.

Put poisons out of reach

Most poisoning accidents involve medicines, household products and cosmetics. Keep all medicines and chemicals out of sight and reach of children, preferably in a locked cupboard. Fit safety catches on your kitchen cupboards and drawers. Be particularly careful about any under-the-sink cupboards, as they tend to contain potentially dangerous cleaning products and sprays, and are at the perfect height for an inquisitive baby.

Be careful of laundry and dishwasher liquitabs too. To a young child, they look like brightly colored sweets and are particularly toxic, and the number of children who have accidentally eaten them has increased in the last few years. They can burn the gullet and some poisoning agents can cause breathing difficulties; seek medical attention immediately if you child has been in contact with them.

Watch out for plants, as children will love to pull off leaves, flowers and berries and some are very poisonous. Dig up (or fence off) any plants with poisonous leaves or berries, such as hydrangea, cyclamen, and lilies.

Pick up choking hazards

Babies and young children are most at risk from choking because they examine the things around them by putting them in their mouths. Children can swallow, inhale or choke on items such as small toys, peanuts, and marbles. Even if you don't leave batteries lying around, they can easily fall out of the TV remote or alarm clock, and watch out for loose coins lying around or on the floor. Choose toys that are suitable for the age of your child. If you have an older child, keep his toys in a separate box or room; toys with small parts are a choking risk to young babies.

Watch out for suffocation risks

All plastic bags pose a suffocation risk to children—even the supermarket bags and shopping bags with holes in. Keep nappy sacks, which are used to dispose of soiled nappies, well out of reach. Not only do they not have holes in them (understandably), they're also made of a flimsier material and don't rustle so they're easily grasped and breathed without parents realizing.

While your baby is little, it's best to keep her apart from any pets. Keep animals, especially cats, away from her sleep areas. No matter how loving your pet, it could suffocate your baby if it decides to lie across him.

Dangers of looped cords

Looped cords such as blind ropes and chains, or curtain tie-backs, can pose a risk to children. About one child in the US dies each month from accidental strangulation on window blind cords. The Consumer Product Safety Commission recommends installing cordless blinds in homes with young children or contacting the Window Covering Safety Council at 800-506-4636 for a free repair kit to make existing blinds safer. If you have an older blind in your home, make sure the cords are well out reach of the most adventurous child, or even better still, removed altogether. Research indicates that most accidental deaths involving blind cords happen in the bedroom and occur in children between 16 and 36 months old. These toddlers are mobile, but their heads still weigh proportionately more than their bodies compared to adults and their muscular control is not yet fully developed, which makes it more difficult for them to free themselves if they become entangled.

In addition, don't hang drawstring bags where a child could get his head through the loop of the drawstring. Do not place your child's crib, bed, playpen, or highchair near a window and keep pull cords on curtains and blinds short and out of reach using cleats, cord tidies, clips or ties. Hide cables and extension leads behind furniture. Remove cords from coats or hoodies too.

Safety around water

A child can drown in less than 1 inch of water, so they should always be under constant supervision when in or near any water. Never leave your child in the bath unsupervised, even for a moment and even if he has an older sibling to watch him. Don't leave uncovered bowls or buckets of water around the home and paddling pools should be emptied and stored away when not in use. If you have a garden pond, it should be securely fenced off (or fill it in while the children are young) and take special care when visiting other people's gardens.

Other potential danger zones

Want to babyproof your coffee table? Stick a soft foam table guard around it to protect your little one from knocks and bangs. Fit corner cushions as sharp edges can be very hazardous for babies and toddlers, especially when they're learning to crawl, pull themselves up, and walk, as they'll be unsteady on their feet. Simply baby-proof all your shelf and furniture edges with corner cushions to avoid accidents. Move valuables and breakables up a level too.

Doors can be dangerous for little fingers (especially the hinge side). You can buy cheap and simple door guards that prevent the door from fully closing so that little hands can't be trapped.

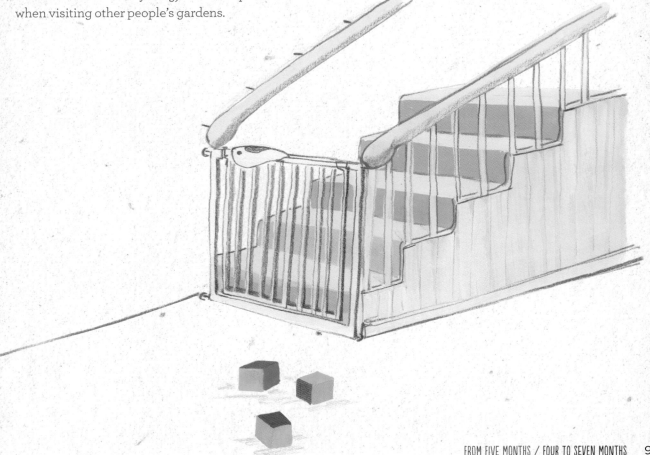

TRAVELING WITH YOUR BABY

If anyone deserves a holiday, it's us moms. But before you start fantasizing about far-flung locations and chic hotels, remember that with a baby or toddler in tow, you also need to put a lot of thought and planning into the details. That way you can all have the calm, relaxing break you've earned.

What type of holiday

While you may have been happy in basic hotels or budget bed and breakfast places when it was just you and your partner, now you have a baby, it's worth thinking again about your accommodation. Hotels may not have kitchen facilities and you may only have one room, so think about what you really need from your space to feel relaxed while you are away. Holiday cottages, villas, or cabins are quite good as they provide your own enclosed space with facilities, but there are other rooms for the adults to relax in once the baby is asleep.

When you go on holiday with your child, chances are you'll spend more time in your accommodation than you did before, especially in the evenings. So think about your priorities when it comes to how much you spend. You may want to head to the beach or have a short trip to town, but with young children, it's easier to have a comfortable base. You'll probably save money in other areas, such as expensive trips out or restaurant dinners.

Think about safety aspects too—this is especially important if you book a long way ahead. Even if your baby isn't particularly mobile when you book, he may be on his feet by the time you leave. If there is a pool check that it is fenced off. If there is a garden, is it secure?

Think about where you want to go

When it comes to location, everybody dreams of white sand beaches and year-round sunshine, but you can get that without having to take a young baby on a long flight with layovers and time-zone changes. If you're happy to go further afield, go for it! Otherwise consider whether you want to look

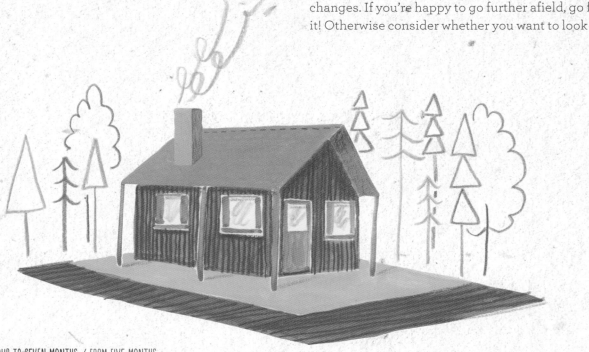

for somewhere nearer home where you can enjoy some sunshine too. Aim for the simplest transfer possible and a short trip to the airport from home—find out where you can fly to from your local airport. The less pre- and post-holiday travel you can do, the better. Once you have arrived consider how you could make the transfer process as smooth as possible. The hotel or villa owner may be able to arrange to collect you, or choose a car hire company that's based at the airport.

Don't worry too much about activities in the area; do as much or as little as feels right. Simple things such as being able to walk to a restaurant, the shops, or the local play area can feel like plenty when you have a young baby. The expensive and tiring activities such as theme parks and castles can be held off until your child is a little older.

Don't underestimate the power of the beach. As long as you're careful on the safety front, picking a holiday location near a beach is great because there's plenty to keep your baby entertained and space for him to move around while you keep an eye on him. Just remember to keep him well protected and stay out of the sun when it's at its strongest (11am to 4pm)—you will need an umbrella and/or some nice shady trees.

What to take with you
Finally, draw up a list of equipment. There is so much stuff you need when you have a baby— bottles, cots, highchairs, strollers, car seats. Sometimes it seems like the list is endless, but draw one up and you can work out what you really need and what might already be available in your holiday accommodation. Ask whether they can supply a high chair, crib, and stair gate for example. If they don't have a piece of equipment that you think you'll need such as a potty, it's always worth asking if they'll be able to provide it.

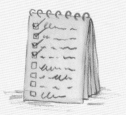

REAL LIFE

·····································

"Being organized is key"

"Going on holiday with baby twins felt like a complete nightmare at first, but I could do it as long as I was completely organized. So I started by making checklists of everything I thought I would need, and then crossed off the stuff I would probably never use. Doing this made me feel in control and ticking things off as I packed them was really satisfying!"

SEEMA, MOM TO TWINS AMBER AND ROSIE, TWO

BABY SWIMMING

In terms of encouraging overall physical development, consider baby swimming lessons. Before a baby learns to crawl, swimming is the only skill requiring him to use his whole body at the same time—this is important for coordination and balance.

EXPERT TIP

IS MY BABY THE RIGHT WEIGHT?
You will have been to get your baby weighed in the early months and know how he has been growing in relation to the weight reference charts in your baby documents. You should still be taking him to be weighed every month (see page 40).
But if you are worried about your baby being underweight or overweight, do talk to your baby's pediatrician to put your mind at rest. He or she will consider your baby's weight as well as his overall health and his appearance and behavior. Is he alert, with good skin color, and muscle tone? The pediatrician will want to know if your baby asks for feeds and is he usually satisfied after them, as well as whether he is peeing and pooing normally—these are all good signs.
If you're ever concerned about any aspect of your baby's development, always contact your baby's pediatrician for advice or a check-up.

PENNY LAZELL
Healthcare professional

Helping your partner and baby to bond

It's just as important for your partner to bond with your baby as it is for you to and, even if you are on maternity leave and he or she is back at work straight after the birth, there are ways that they can strengthen their emotional ties with your little one.

Keeping in touch during the day
If your partner is concerned about missing out on time with your baby when he is at the office and you are still at home, try keeping in touch during the day—perhaps plan to Facetime him with your baby at lunchtime, so it won't interrupt his work, and/or send him photos or videos of your little one at other times.

Involve him in activies when he's home
Bear in mind that, after being out of the new baby house for most of the day, it might be hard for your partner to come back, see your lovely bond and have to break into the "coupledom" that you and your baby have created together. You may also find that from seven or so months, your baby may show a clear preference to be with you and so now is the time to get them to know each other a little better. Time and effort during the early months will lay the foundations for them to have a good relationship when the baby is older.

Keep special tasks for him

Of course, doing some of the practical side of things is all part of shared parenting, so your partner can give your baby his evening bath or bedtime bottle; these everyday, precious experiences will bring them closer and make him feel needed and included.

Let him prepare his own routines

It's a good idea for your partner to schedule in "baby time" into his day and create little routines of his own too, such as singing a certain song, sharing a certain book, or just making up a story, every time he's home. Just making time to play with the baby every day will help the father/baby bond strengthen. These routines will become familiar to your baby and will help them to connect with each other.

Give him time

The other thing to remember is that you are now the "expert" parent as you have spent the most hours with your little one, so be patient with your partner if he is not as responsive to your baby (or as good at bathtime) as you are. Show him what you do, or just leave him to have fun with your baby. He does not have to do everything the same way as you. It's another way for him to strengthen his bond with your baby.

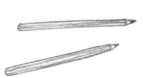

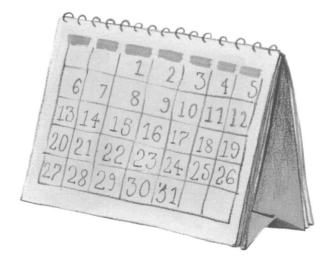

CHAPTER NINE
FROM SIX MONTHS

Now it is time for the next big change: introducing solid foods into you baby's diet. Over the next few months you'll be cutting your baby's milk feeds down (slowly) to three feeds a day—one in the morning, one before bed, and one in between. From now your baby should be napping for just under three hours a day.

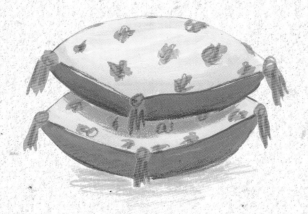

NEW VIEW OF THE WORLD

Between now and eight months, your little one may be sitting without support. At first, sit her on the floor propped up with cushions in case she wobbles, and put her favorite toys beside her to encourage her to turn. As her neck and trunk muscles strengthen she'll adapt to her new upright view and she won't need the cushions any more. If your baby is not able to sit unsupported by nine months, talk to your pediatrician.

Your baby may start crawling or bum-shuffling soon, although some babies don't crawl until after their first birthday. There are also babies who don't crawl at all—they go straight to walking.

QUICK FIX

SAFE SLEEPING

As soon as your baby can sit up, put the cot mattress down to its lowest level to make sure your baby is safe.

EXPERT TIP

NOT SLEEPING THROUGH THE NIGHT?

If you are having trouble settling your baby or she's wants a feed at night, try to forget about how she "should be sleeping" and focus on what works for you. Try to enjoy the sleepy snuggles and night feeds when it's just you and her—they won't last for long. Take it day by day, and things will improve. It helps if your baby learns to fall asleep without you in the room. Try my "softly softly" method; the key to making it work is to be totally repetitive. Dim the lights, pull the curtains, keep everything boring. Choose a low-key soothing method that calms your baby: hold her hands, make shush-shush sounds, play white noise, or quietly say "sleepy time," then gradually leave the room. Wait it out. This can take four weeks or even longer and you will probably question whether it's having any effect. But if you stick with it, your hard work will suddenly kick in one night.

TINA SOUTHWOOD
Sleep consultant

INTRODUCING SOLID FOODS

By six months, you'll start your baby on tiny amounts of "solid" (well-cooked and puréed) vegetables, fruit, or powdered food such as baby rice, which is mixed with milk. The idea is to start her on the road to real food by introducing to her different tastes and textures while continuing her normal milk feeds. You've got the bibs, bowls, and blender all ready, so when's the right time?

The best time to begin

The official guideline is to wait until your baby is 26 weeks old. Health experts argue that before this your baby's digestive system is still developing and introducing solids could increase the risk of infections and allergies. There's also the argument that your baby should be exclusively breastfed until six months old, so solids would get in the way of this. In reality, the real danger is giving your baby solids when your baby's stomach lining and the enzymes needed for digestion aren't yet developed.

You don't have to start solids at exactly six months. Your baby does need to be able to coordinate the small hand movements and have developed the tongue thrust needed for swallowing. This often happens around the six-month mark, but it can be earlier. Often moms start to give solids earlier because milk no longer seems to be filling their baby up (although she should continue with milk feeds). But your baby being hungry isn't alone a sign to switch on the blender. If your baby is suddenly hungry all the time, or she's waking during the night, it's worth remembering babies often go through a growth spurt at around four months. It may seem like she needs solids to stay satisfied, but she may not be ready. Always check with baby's pediatrician for advice on whether you should start solids earlier than six months. The very earliest that you can start solids is four months, and protein should not be introduced before six months, so if you are starting solids early, stick to baby rice and fruit and veg. It's a good idea to attend a baby first aid course, especially before you start solids. The course will tell you how to treat choking as well as other potential emergencies.

EXPERT TIP

IS SHE READY FOR SOLIDS?
Your baby may be ready to start trying out solid food if:
- she can sit up by herself in her high chair
- she can hold her head steady and turn her head easily
- she can coordinate her eyes, hands, and mouth so that she is able to look at the food, pick it up, and would also be able to put it to her mouth by herself
- she doesn't push food back out of her mouth

DR REBECCA CHICOT
Child development and parenting expert

YOUR BABY'S FIRST FOODS

Every baby is different and while some enjoy trying new tastes, and move through solids quickly and easily, others may need a little more time and support from parents to get used to new textures. However, there are some general tips for babies being introduced to solids at six months from Registered Nutritionist Charlotte Stirling-Reed that can help make it easier for both of you.

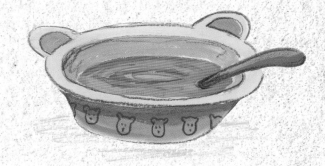

First foods and purées

Moving from milk to proper solids is a big jump, so the best first foods for your baby are well-cooked vegetables and fruit (one taste at a time initially), which are puréed, if you are using the traditional method for solids. Keep the texture nice and smooth and not too dissimilar to milk yet to allow your baby to get used to new flavors and a new way of feeding. If starting your baby with purées, you really only need to offer them for up to a few weeks before gently encouraging her to move on to textured foods, although there's no one-size-fits-all rule.

It's a good idea to focus on vegetables initially and not just fruit. Babies are born with a preference for sweet foods and so they won't need much encouragement to enjoy fruit. However, it may take a few tries for a baby to like different vegetable tastes, especially the more bitter green vegetables. Keep trying though and offer variety, as familiarity will help your baby learn to like these new tastes, especially if she doesn't like them initially. Combining favorite flavors with new ones, for example sweet potato and chicken, is a good way to introduce more new tastes.

Baby-led solids

Alternatively, you may want to try baby-led solids, which is when you skip the purée stage and let your baby pick up and eat soft foods herself from the start. If practising this sit with your baby all the time she is feeding to reduce the risk of choking.

Mix and match

A combination of the two methods can often be a good way to get your baby onto solids. You can offer her puréed foods initially, but put some soft finger foods on her highchair tray at the same time to encourage self-feeding.

DID YOU KNOW?

. . . .

The American Academy of Pediatrics recommends that all breastfed babies are given 400IU of vitamin D oral drops until they are drinking 17fl oz of cow's milk (not before age one) or baby formula. Babies who have 17fl oz of formula per day don't need the drops since most formula is fortified with vitamin D.

CHARLOTTE STIRLING-REED'S 5 STEPS

Choose a time for the first feed when you are both relaxed and alert. Try in the middle of a milk feed so your baby isn't too hungry or full either.

1 Start simply

Begin with baby rice mixed with her usual milk. Offer a little bit on the tip of a shallow baby spoon. Be prepared for it to come dribbling out or for her to pull strange faces while she works out what to do with it. Don't expect her to take more than a couple of spoonfuls at the first meals. This stage is to get your baby used to taking food, training her to manipulate her tongue and move food around her mouth. For baby-led solids try very soft things like banana or avocado slices.

2 Be patient

Try not to get frustrated when your baby rejects a food—research suggests it may take her up to 10 tastes (on different days) to learn to like it. It's important to set a good example, so eat with your baby and let her see you enjoy a variety of foods. If she refuses something, don't force it, just move on to something else and try it again in a week or so. If a particular taste is rejected, you could try combining it with a favorite one at another meal.

3 Choose the right ingredients

If you choose to start solids before six months, it's best to begin with cereals (rice, oatmeal, or barley), vegetables or fruit. Introduce one ingredient at a time every two to three days; if she has a reaction to something, you'll know what it is. Avoid honey until she is at least a year old because it's linked to botulism. You may gradually introduce yogurt or cheese, but don't give cow's milk as a drink until your baby is 12 months old, because it doesn't have the right nutrition profile for babies. Eggs can be eaten after she's six months old, but only if they are very well cooked through to avoid a salmonella risk. Avoid anything large such as whole grapes as they pose a serious choking risk. Avoid sugary foods and don't add salt when preparing your baby's meals. Never leave your baby alone while she is eating

4 Prepare to get messy

Cheeks smeared with sauce and lumps of banana in her hair will be a common sight. When babies are born their skin is extremely sensitive to touch. Your baby needs to experience different textures and sensations on her skin and hands during meals to help desensitize her and make her feel comfortable around food. If you're constantly wiping her face and worrying that she's dipped her hands in her yoghurt, she could grow up with a fear of new foods and textures and turn into a fussy eater. Put down a splash mat (or newspaper) and invest in a coverall bib if you're worried about the mess. Instead grab your camera—those first photographs with solids are a baby album classic.

5 Keep it safe

Prepare your baby's food carefully because her immune system is still developing. Wash your hands before you prepare food. Wash cutlery or bowls in hot soapy water or a dishwasher.

Make sure you wash all fruit and vegetables and peel if necessary to remove dirt that could cause illness. When cooking food for your baby, make sure it's cooked thoroughly, especially eggs (up to one year), fish, and meat. Your baby can't eat food as hot as your meals, so let hers cool slightly before feeding it to her. Always throw away leftover baby food. Reheating it will only lead to bacteria multiplying, potentially giving your baby a tummy upset. If you serve store-bought baby food, spoon a small portion from the jar into a bowl to avoid waste. If your baby doesn't finish the jar, and you've put the spoon from her mouth into the container, you'd have to throw it out.

Q&A WITH CHARLOTTE STIRLING-REED
NUTRITIONIST

"Do I need to reduce my 6 month baby's formula milk feeds during when starting solids?"

"When you first start solids, your baby will continue to have the same number of milk feeds and should still be getting 17½ to 21fl oz of milk per day plus one meal of solid food. As you increase the amount of food, you'll find her appetite for milk reduces and you can drop a milk feed. She should be on three meals a day a month after starting solids. By 12 months reduce her milk intake to a maximom of around 10½ to 12½fl oz."

"How will I know if my baby is allergic to a food?"

"If you have a family history talk to your doctor before you start solids. If your baby is sensitive to a particular food she may start coughing, have a runny nose, or a rash, or eczema may appear. Other symptoms to watch for include diarrhea, vomiting, wheezing, and sore or red eyes. Foods with known allergens, include nuts, cow's milk, eggs, shellfish, cereals, and soy. Never diagnose an allergy yourself. Only a doctor can confirm as symptoms could relate to an illness that needs attention."

"How can I tell if my baby's full?"

"Look out for the same signals you've learned to read when your baby has had enough milk. If you're worried about whether your baby is eating too much or too little, take her to the doctor's office to be weighed. At six or seven months, a baby's weight gain slows anyway, particularly once she starts moving more, but if she jumps up or down a centile, then your pediatrician can give you advice."

"How do I switch my baby to a cup?"

"The key is to get a cup that encourages sipping rather than sucking. Fill a free-flow beaker without a valve with water and give it to your baby at meals or between milk feeds. Cups with handles are easier for her to grasp. Once she's used to sipping from a free-flow beaker, gradually switch it to an open cup. Don't put too much liquid in the cup, so it won't matter if she spills it. Sipping develops the muscles around her mouth and lips, which in turn helps with speech development. By the time your baby is 12 months, she should have stopped using a bottle with a teat. If she continues after that she'll associate it with comfort, especially if she goes to sleep with a bottle, and this can be a difficult habit to break."

SOLIDS AT 6 MONTHS

You could offer purées for anything from a few days to a couple of weeks. Try mashed foods when she's ready, then, once she's used to the texture, try chopped, cooked, or soft food. Using purées for too long could impact on development. Every baby is different so talk to your pediatrician if necessary.

CHARLOTTE STIRLING-REED
Nutritionist

If she's eating purées:

Phase one
Choose two or three out of: cooked sweet potato, broccoli or pear purée, baby porridge, avocado, and banana

Phase two
puréed cooked chicken and broccoli, mashed potato

Phase three
cooked and mashed butternut squash, apple, and very ripe peeled pear (no more purée)

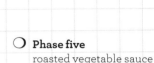

Phase four
boiled and mashed lamb and carrot

Phase five
roasted vegetable sauce with baby pasta

Phase six
scrambled eggs, lightly toasted bread fingers

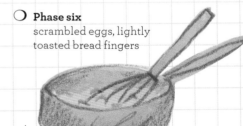

EMBRACING BABY MESS

The time has come for you to really embrace domestic chaos (if you haven't already). Don't stress—it's part of being a parent!

Daily life with babies and children goes hand in hand with a bit (ok, sometimes a lot) of mess. Parents are entitled to do as much or as little towards the housework as they want, whether that means letting the house become messy, paying someone else to help with the cleaning, or doing it together at the weekend. We're playing more with our kids too and that often takes priority. It's a healthy attitude to have and we can only gain from it.

Twitter and Facebook both have many mom members who post pictures of their overflowing cupboards and write about their messy living

If she's baby-led:

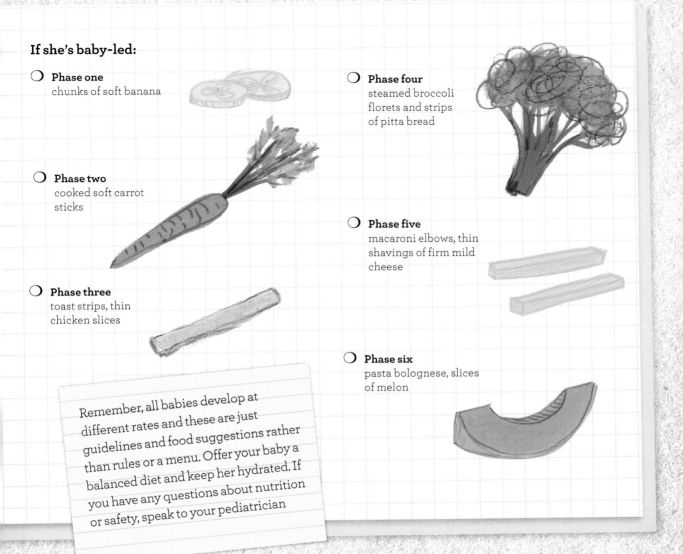

○ **Phase one**
chunks of soft banana

○ **Phase two**
cooked soft carrot sticks

○ **Phase three**
toast strips, thin chicken slices

○ **Phase four**
steamed broccoli florets and strips of pitta bread

○ **Phase five**
macaroni elbows, thin shavings of firm mild cheese

○ **Phase six**
pasta bolognese, slices of melon

Remember, all babies develop at different rates and these are just guidelines and food suggestions rather than rules or a menu. Offer your baby a balanced diet and keep her hydrated. If you have any questions about nutrition or safety, speak to your pediatrician

rooms. This new trend for honesty about how our homes really look is something to celebrate. It's OK to enjoy normality and the real, flawed chaos that emerges when you're a parent. Tensions are only likely to develop if your partner has different (higher) standards than you or vice versa. But if they're unhappy with certain things not being done, it's up to them to take on the responsibility for doing them.

Of course, we're not suggesting you live in an unhealthy house. It's about prioritizing, finding shortcuts, and ditching ideals. Your physical surroundings can affect your mental state. So, if the state of your home is making you feel anxious, then you need to have a quick clear up. Otherwise, it's a question of finding a happy balance for you and your baby.

Managing your new anxieties

Your newborn was a handful. At three months, you were still exhausted. By six months, you still haven't cracked it and you've got squashed banana in your hair? All of this totally normal.

Research shows that by the time a baby is six months old, two thirds of moms are struggling, and one in six don't begin to enjoy their babies properly until after their first birthday. With a newborn, you have attention and visits from well-wishers, friends, and relatives. But, six months later, fewer people ask how you are, or visit, and the day-to-day reality of being at home with a baby kicks in. To add to this, your baby's sleep often regresses around now, either because she's ready for solids, she's teething, or she's just increasingly mobile. Although you may be getting more sleep than you did in those first few weeks, the previous months will still be taking their toll.

Your hormones are changing

The build-up of exhaustion, both physical and mental, can trigger slumps in mood around six months after birth. If you've recently stopped or cut down on breastfeeding, there's also a scientific reason behind a six-month low as it prompts a change in hormone levels.

When breastfeeding stops, oxytocin (which has an anti-anxiety effect) levels drop as the hormone is no longer needed for lactation. Many women report feeling uptight and anxious as a result. Even cutting back on feeds, as your baby moves to solids, can trigger symptoms. On top of the hormones and tiredness, there's a dawning sense that you can no longer put your life on hold (and live in that new baby bubble) and it becomes decision time. It's common to find yourself facing big questions about your life and your future as a family, which can add to the anxiety.

Start looking forwards

By the time your baby is six months old, she has usually developed enough to enable you to start

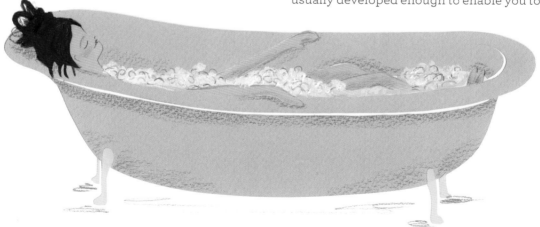

thinking of yourself a bit more. It's a brilliant time to take stock and consider your future, but equally it can all be too much if you're not mentally prepared for this new phase. If you worry, try to channel your thoughts in a constructive way. Set aside time every week to tackle tasks such as looking into baby-proofing the living room, but don't let them dominate life.

Try to identify specific problems that are getting you down, and don't let them overwhelm you. For example, your career might be a source of concern and you'd feel better after a chat with your boss, or half an hour online considering other options. Most importantly, rather than beating yourself up about not being totally on top of things, cut yourself some slack. A mom of a six month old needs to look after herself just as much as a mom of a six week old. For the last half year, you will have been so busy nurturing your baby that you may have forgotten to look after yourself. It's really important that you eat well, get plenty of rest, and recharge your batteries whenever you can.

Deal with your feelings head-on. Talk to your partner. Get regular fresh air and socialize more if necessary. Make sure you have an activity booked in at least once a day, so you get out of the house. If you don't know where to start, check with your town's parks and recreation department, which may have information on mom-and-baby groups or talk to the pediatrician. As your baby starts to sleep better, you both get the hang of solids, and your hormones settle, you'll be able to deal with things more easily.

EXPERT TIP

ACCEPTING SUPPORT

For moms caught up in the perfect storm of cumulative tiredness, hormonal havoc, and high expectations, finding support should be a priority. Whether you turn to friends, family, your doctor or yur baby's pediatrician, the first step to overcoming a difficult period is admitting you're having one. If it threatens to become more serious, for example, you persistently feel sad, fatigued, irritable or can't enjoy anything, including your baby, make sure your doctor or a therapist rules out postpartum depression. Sometimes a proper diagnosis is missed in the turmoil of birth and the early days with a baby.

MIA SCOTLAND
Clinical psychologist

CHAPTER TEN
FROM SEVEN MONTHS

Your baby is about to embark on another new phase: crawling, although this can start anywhere between six and nine months. His stomach, shoulder, neck, and arm muscles are also getting stronger by the day as he rolls, reaches, and grabs for things. About now he will start to balance on his hands and knees. Eventually he will push off to move around—you may be surprised at how quickly he will master it.

ENCOURAGING YOUR BABY TO START MOVING

The new phase in your baby's development will start with a form of crawling—essentially when he learns to balance on his hands and knees and then push off to move around. Crawling encourages the opposite sides of the body to work together, and trains hand-eye coordination, which is also useful for tasks such as self-feeding. When he starts to show interest in crawling you can help him by laying him over a cushion, so his knees and hands are on the floor. Place a favorite toy (or yourself) just out of reach to encourage him to move towards it.

Babies start crawling in a number of different ways. About half of all babies begin by shimmying along on their stomachs using their elbows to propel themselves forward. If sitting upright a bottom crawler pushes his hands on the floor to his sides and scoots his but along the floor; some babies start off crawling backwards. Don't worry if he shows no interest in crawling though—some babies don't do it at all—and go straight to walking.

What else can he do now?
He loves to look at picture books, and can now begin to feed himself too. His legs are getting stronger and its won't be too long before he starts to pull himself up onto his feet (see page 127).

Safety first
As soon as your baby can crawl (or better still, before he starts), install safety gates at the top and bottom of your stairs to stop him climbing up and/or falling down them. Also fit safety catches to cupboards to keep their contents out of reach, and devices to prevent your interior doors from closing (find out more about baby-proofing on

EXPERT TIP

STARTING TO PULL HIMSELF UP
Just as he started to crawl, keen for a better view of the world, you'll probably find your baby hanging onto the furniture next as he tries to pull himself up. Strength in his upper and lower body is needed here, along with coordination. Later he'll also use these skills for cruising—the side-stepping motion he makes while holding onto the couch for support.

Make sure there are safe things for your baby to pull up on and be there to comfort him when he falls back down with a bump. He may even be tempted to climb—so make sure low furniture is kept away from windows and that windows are fitted with locks or safety catches.

DR REBECCA CHICOT
Child development and parenting expert

page 93). In addition, never leave your baby alone and watch him when he is crawling around your home to avoid accidents—babies can move fast once they get going.

EXPERT TIP

....

HE CAN STAND IN HIS COT

From the age of seven months, your baby may well master a new skill: pulling himself upright in his crib (make sure the mattress is at its lowest possible position now). What many parents then discover is that while their baby is good at pulling himself up, he can't actually get back down again. Once he's stuck in the upright position, he'll start crying for you. The solution is to spend lots of time during the day letting your baby pull himself upright on your furniture and then showing him how to plop back down onto a cushion.

TINA SOUTHWOOD
Sleep consultant

ILLNESS IN THE FIRST YEAR

When you know how annoying and uncomfortable coughs, blocked noses, and sore throats can be, it's even harder to watch your baby struggling with one. Babies suffer from lots of coughs and colds because their immune systems are less developed than ours; the good news is that for each one they have they are developing more antibodies.

Coughs and colds are usually caused by viruses, and will usually clear up on their own within a week or so. During this time, it's about treating the symptoms to keep your baby comfortable with rest and plenty of fluids. Keep an eye on how much he's drinking and how wet his nappies are. Stay calm and reassure him if he's distressed. Ring your baby's pediatrician straight away if your child's breathing appears to be difficult, the fever does not come down after giving him infant acetaminophen or ibuprofen, or you have other concerns. Occasionally a secondary bacterial infection can develop from a cold.

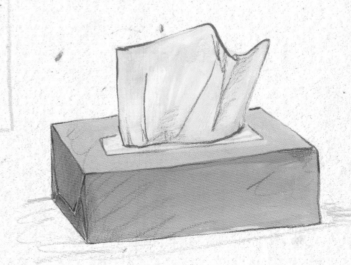

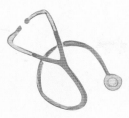

REAL LIFE

"I always go with my gut instinct"

"I've always been a worrier, but when it comes to my baby's health, I never feel silly about asking the pediatrician if I'm concerned about her. When she was a month old I noticed her breathing was a little fast and took her straight to the pediatrician. It turned out that she had a common infection called bronchiolitis, which I had never heard of. I'm glad I didn't wait before getting her treated."

JANE, MOM TO OLIVIA, ONE

DID YOU KNOW?

If you are giving a baby infant acetaminophen or ibuprofen, never exceed the stated dose and don't medicate a baby under the age of three months unless your pediatrician advises it. Don't give both unless advised to do so by the doctor.

Q&A

"How can I tell whether my baby is constipated and what you can I do to help him?"

Family doctor **PHILIPPA KAYE** says, "Your baby could be constipated if he is not passing poo as often as he usually does, he is distressed or seems uncomfortable or straining to open his bowels, and produces small, hard, pellet-like poo. Babies on formula are also more likely to become constipated than breastfed ones because formula milk is harder to digest. Constipation could be down to dehydration and introducing solids or new foods can cause it while your baby's body learns how to manage the change.

"If your child is breastfed, he may need more breast milk. However, formula-fed babies may need some extra cooled boiled water. Don't dilute his milk, but offer water as an extra between milk feeds. If your baby's on solids, give him plenty of water and perhaps a small amount of diluted fruit juice. If these remedies don't work, see your baby's pediatrician."

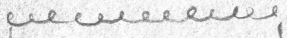

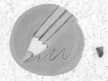

EXPERT TIP

• •

WHEN IS IT SERIOUS?

Call your pediatrician urgently or take your child to the hospital if you notice any of the following:

• high-pitched, weak or continuous cries
• lack of responsiveness, marked slowdown or increased floppiness
• bulging fontanelle (the soft spot on a baby's head)
• neck stiffness in an older child
• no drinking for more than eight hours
• temperature higher 100.4°F for a baby under three months, or over 102.2°F for ages three to six months
• high temperature, but cold feet and hands
• high temperature, with quietness and listlessness despite being given infant acetaminophen or ibuprofen
• seizures
• blue, very pale, mottled or gray skin
• unusually drowsy, hard to wake up or doesn't seem to recognize you
• unable to stay awake, even when awoken
• repeated or bile-stained vomiting

DR PHILIPPA KAYE
Family doctor

YOUR FAMILY FIRST AID KIT

Keep a box of adhesive bandage strips and essential medications at home. Keep it in a cool dry place and well out of the way of children. Always check the age advice on the packet as some medicines are not suitable for young babies.

● **Thermometer**
Keep track of your baby's temperature with a thermometer. The quickest and easiest to use is a digital ear thermometer; it gives a result in seconds. In children under five, a fever is considered to be a temperature higher than 99.5°F.

● **Pain and fever relief**
Keep some adult pain relief on hand for your own headaches, period pain or backache. Infant acetaminophen or infant ibuprofen is also useful for bringing down fevers in your baby—always read the packet instructions and check the correct dose for your child's age. Avoid ibuprofen if your child has asthma, unless advised by your family doctor.

● **Adhesive bandage strips**
Whether it's to protect a grazed knee or a painful cut, bandage strips from your medicine cabinet will always help to make your child feel better. Even more so if they feature their favorite TV characters.

● **Sterile gauze pads**
Used to clean around a dirty wound.

● **Sterile dressings**
Use these to cover bigger cuts and grazes. You may want to take your baby or toddler to the pediatrician to have him looked at.

● **Antiseptic**
Apply antiseptic lotion or cream to cuts and grazes to protect against any infection-causing bacteria. It also works on bites and stings.

- **Diaper/barrier cream**
  Soothe painful diaper rash and prevent redness on your baby's skin with a barrier cream.
- **Oral rehydration solution (Pedialyte)**
  If you or your baby has diarrhoea, it's important to replace lost fluids, body salts, and glucose. Pedialyte comes in liquid or powder form and aids rehydration. Always consult your baby's pediatrician if he has a bout of diarrhea.
- **Colic drops**
  In some instances colic can be eased by special drops containing simeticone or lactase.
- **Antihistamine**
  Help ease itchy skin from irritants or things your baby is allergic to with antihistamine ointment.
- **Heartburn relief**
  You can buy infant indigestion medication to help reflux (see page 36). Get advice from your doctor or pharmacist before giving it to your baby.
- **Teething gel**
  Helps ease your baby's gum pain when teething.
- **Cotton balls**
  Useful for early diaper changes, or cleaning the eyes if your baby has conjunctivitis.
- **Sun cream**
  Protecting your baby's skin from the sun is vital. Keep suncream to hand at all times of the year, just in case there's an odd unseasonally hot day (it does happen). Try an SPF50+ lotion made for kids that will cater for sensitive young skin.
- **Medicine dispenser**
  If giving your baby medicine has turned into a messy splatterfest because he wriggles so much, try using a medicine dispenser. It works like a syringe and comes with children's medicines. You can also buy varieties with a dummy attachment that enables your baby to suck the medicine.
- **Nasal aspirator**
  Babies and children can't blow their noses,

so if your little one is bunged up, a nasal aspirator, which works to suck mucus out of your baby's nose (yep, delightful), can be useful.
- **Tweezers**
  Handy for pulling splinters out of fingers.
- **Emery board**
  Useful for filing a young baby's nails.

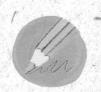

EXPERT TIP

CALL AN AMBULANCE IMMEDIATELY IF:
- there's a spotty, purple-red rash anywhere on the body that does not fade if pressed, for example, the rash is still visible when a clear glass is pressed on it (this could be a sign of meningitis or septicaemia)
- your baby has difficulty breathing, fast breathing, grunting while breathing, or if your child is working hard to breathe—for example, sucking his stomach in under their ribs (call an ambulance if you baby if struggling for breath)
- severe abdominal pain
- your child is unresponsive

DR PHILIPPA KAYE
Family doctor

How to be you with a baby

Yes, you're in a completely different headspace when you have a baby—but that doesn't mean the old you is gone. It's just about making time to still enjoy the things you love.

Schedule spontaneity

You used to love a last-minute film, but having a baby can mean everything needs more planning. So, do just that—plan spontaneous time. Ask if your partner or a relative can sit for a few hours so you're not worrying about your baby, then do whatever you want. Just give yourself the headspace to relax.

Show your relationship some love

Your couple priorities change with this little person you've both made, but you still need to create time for each other. It's being a couple that got you here, so eat together, or have a night on the sofa where you can chat once a week. Embrace the little, easy things that make you both feel loved.

Pick your battles

If having everything tidy and in order is your thing, then your baby world will have turned your house upside down. Breathe. Now, pick three easy things to prioritize or reorder, then you can feel more chilled about the ones that are harder to control. Try, for example, always putting the TV remote in the same place or making sure your own bedroom's tidy, even though the lounge room is toy central, then choose one more.

Boost your self-confidence

If you're missing your usual interests, whether it is fashion, music, reading, or sport, don't cut them out of your new life. Yes, you have new priorities, but it's important to indulge the parts of yourself that aren't about motherhood, too. It could be doing your nails or playing your favorite CD while you get ready for your baby yoga class. Bring what you love into your new routine.

Adapt your friendships

When you have a baby, it's natural to worry about your social dynamic changing, especially if you're the first of your friends to do it. But that doesn't mean things ending; it can be a new beginning. Be open to a new social circle at mom and baby classes or in the park, so you have people who understand this new stage too. But make time for your other friends and the connections you have that make you feel like "you." Ask them to come round to yours at first if it's easier, the chances are they'll love a cuddle with your baby.

NOTES

You're getting to know your baby better each day, but things are about to get really interesting as he's moving around more and more!

4 TO 7 MONTHS

MONTH 4

Your baby could even show signs of teething around now and you can sometimes feel red swollen lumps under her gums as her teeth break through. Some babies also experience diarrhea and a sore bottom around this time but it's disputed if this is a direct effect of teething. Remember, it is absolutely fine if teeth don't appear this early on.

She's becoming increasingly mobile so think about baby-proofing your home sooner rather than later to be on the safe side.

MONTH 5

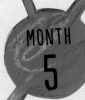

MONTH 5

Start brushing her teeth as soon as they erupt and try making a game of it to keep it fun.

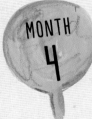

MONTH 4

MONTH 4

Your baby will start babbling more now and could copy simple movements.

Her strength is improving all the time, encourage it to keep on building with regular tummy time.

She'll soon be able to roll over, sometimes at night, so lots of tummy time is important during the day to encourage her to build strength.

Your baby's muscles are still building up and she may almost be able to sit up by herself for very short periods.

MONTH 6

MONTH 6

Keep encouraging strength building through tummy time and baby swimmning classes.

Make sure you lower her mattress as soon as she can sit up to keep your baby safe in her crib.

Your baby could start crawling or bum-shuffling very soon.

MONTH 7

With all this exploring, and because her immune system is still developing, your baby will be getting coughs and colds throughout her first year. This is something that will get better with time.

She will soon be able to pull herself up independently but will still need help getting back to sitting—give her plenty of practice during the day when you can keep an eye on her.

MONTH 7

MONTH 7

MONTH 6

You can start solids around now—look out for the signs that show she's physically ready.

Encourage her to keep moving by placing a favorite toy or book just out of reach.

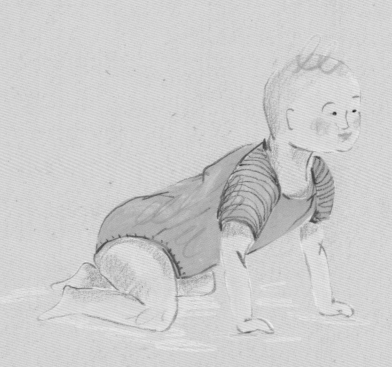

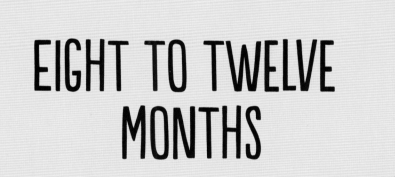

EIGHT TO TWELVE MONTHS

CHAPTER ELEVEN
FROM EIGHT MONTHS

Between now and the end of her first year, your baby
will pass another milestone: developing a pincer grip,
picking up small objects between her thumb and
forefinger. Offering different finger foods, cooked
peas or pasta, can help her refine this skill. Make sure
the foods are age-appropriate (to prevent choking)
and stay close at all times just in case. Read brightly
colored picture books to her too and encourage her to
turn the pages herself.

ENCOURAGING HER DEVELOPMENT

As you continue to see your baby's character develop, now is a great time to start introducing her to positive traits, such as patience. Your baby will probably be indicating what she wants with gestures, but hold off for 15 seconds or so before giving her the toy she wants. Tell her in a calm voice that you're just going to wait a moment. By doing this, you're teaching her about patience and also to trust that you will answer her needs. If your baby is not crawling by now you should talk to your baby's pediatrician.

SEPARATION ANXIETY

You may also be contending with a new, slightly more difficult issue that means you'll be her number one person even more than usual.

For months, your baby has been happy to be held by anyone, then suddenly her cries make it clear the only person she wants is you. Welcome to separation anxiety. You've finally got your baby's sleep routine sorted—but now she's started waking up and crying for no reason at all, and she hates being left alone too. It's all very confusing for everyone.

Separation anxiety, which is a completely normal development milestone, shows just how amazing the bond between you and your baby has become. This huge developmental change occurs from roughly eight to 18 months, but it can start as early as six months. Separation anxiety then tends to wax and wane when babies become toddlers. It might decrease after a baby's first birthday and return around her second birthday, but the patterns can be different from child to child and can be a response to their environment.

Problems at night

It's really common for a baby with separation anxiety to wake more than usual during the night—and struggle to go back to sleep unless she's with you, even if she was sleeping through until now. Your baby may also struggle to fall asleep, even when you stick to the bath and bedtime routine that's always worked up to now.

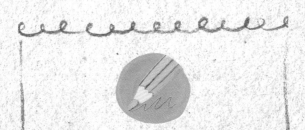

EXPERT TIP

UNDERSTANDING SEPARATION ANXIETY
Separation anxiety is a sign that your baby recognizes you are a separate person. Don't try to force her independence; it won't help if you leave her alone for any length of time at this age. You may notice she isn't just upset when you're not around, but will generally be a lot clingier when you are there. None of this will last forever. Separation anxiety is a normal stage of development and it is also transient; within a few months things will naturally get easier without you actually doing anything special.

DR REBECCA CHICOT
Child development and parenting expert

By day

You may have difficulty dropping your baby off at the daycare center or with the in-home daycare, even when she's been fine with this up to now. This is common, and she may be unhappy going to other people, even her dad. If your little one suddenly goes off her favorite toys, don't despair—this is also really common. You may find she's no longer happy to play alone, even with toys that she previously loved, and she'll cry if you leave her alone, even if it's only for a minute or two. She'll probably want you to play with her, which can be time-consuming for you, but is a great way to reassure her that you're not going anywhere.

It's a good sign

Remind yourself that as exhausting as this is, it means that your child has a good attachment with you and this is a strong psychological sign that she will grow to be confident and independent.

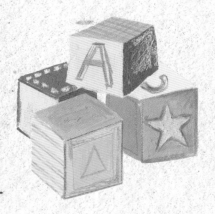

Your post-baby body is better than you think

You may feel exhausted, stressed and less than your best when you've been up half the night with a young baby—but your body could be healthier than you imagine right now.

Benefiting from healthy life changes

When you were pregnant, chances are you overhauled your lifestyle choices to ensure your growing baby got all the best nutrients she could. So, if you've made positive health changes such as quitting smoking and drinking, and cutting down on caffeine plus eating more vitamin-rich foods, these habits will often stick with you once your baby is born. Plus, running around after your little one is probably keeping you fitter than you imagine.

Pregnancy helps your body

You probably enjoyed not having to worry about periods during your pregnancy, but the gynecological health positives can continue after birth, as you could have fewer period cramps. Some women even find that menstrual pain stops altogether after pregnancy and childbirth. Research published in the British Medical Journal has found that childbirth eliminates some of the prostaglandin receptor sites in the uterus. Prostaglandins, the hormones that make the uterus contract during labor, also play a role in monthly menstrual pain. The upshot? Fewer pain-receptor sites means fewer cramps.

Breastfeeding makes you feel good too

If you breastfeed some experts believe it could possibly help to lower your risk of heart disease, Type 2 diabetes and high blood pressure, depending on the length of time you breastfeed for in total. Researchers at Northwestern University, Evanston, say the effect isn't just from helping to shed those post-pregnancy pounds, which can be a side-effect of breastfeeding, it is because the oxytocin released during nursing has heart-healthy properties.

Plus, you're likely to feel surges of love and other good feelings whenever you hold or nurse your little one. A 2011 study from Stanford University found that this emotional surge is thanks to the hormone oxytocin, which plays a big role during the bonding process. But oxytocin is so powerful that one dose can also fend off anxiety for hours and even days.

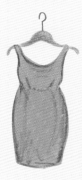

REAL LIFE

"I'm proud of my baby belly"

"Having had two kids, I sometimes feel self-conscious about my body. After carrying two babies my tummy is pretty saggy and my breasts are not what they once were. But you know what? I'm proud of what my body has achieved! I refuse to feel bad about myself when my body has produced such incredible children, and I wouldn't change a thing."
DELLA, MOM TO MILLIE, TWO AND JOSEPHINE, FOUR

CHAPTER TWELVE
FROM NINE MONTHS

From nine to twelve months, your baby needs three milk feeds and three meals a day. He may be sleeping through at night and will have around two hours and 15 minutes sleep during the day. He will also be able let go of things or hand an object to someone on purpose. You can play games to encourage him by giving him toys and asking for them back.

LITTLE CRUISER ON THE GO

Soon your baby will probably have developed his motor skills sufficiently to move around holding on to the furniture. This can be any time between eight and 11 months and it's one of the last steps towards independent walking. Try placing a few chairs in a line, sit him at one end to pull himself up, then sit at the other end with his favorite toy.

LEARNING TO CHEW

Chewing and developing speech use many of the same muscles. Pull faces to make him laugh. He can cope with lumpier food textures, but you may notice him gagging on certain things. This is a natural defence and an essential part of learning to chew. While you should supervise him closely, don't be too alarmed by this (as long as you can see he is able to breathe). Make sure you are aware of how to deal with choking, don't push him to eat more than he wants or if he's not ready. Gently persevere with soft, lumpier foods, and offer finger foods that he can easily manage to chew; with practice he'll control the reflex better. His gums will get firmer and when his teeth break through, chewing becomes easier. If you're worried, talk to your baby's pediatrician.

DID YOU KNOW?

At around nine months your baby begins to demonstrate problem-solving, trial and error, and reasoning skills. Help him along with toys that need a bit of brainwork.

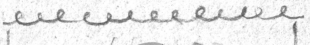

EXPERT TIP

BABY SAYS "MOM" AND "DAD"

There's no prouder moment than when your baby utters her first "mom" or "dad." At five to seven months your baby's vocal cords will be more developed and he'll experiment with different words and sound patterns. This babbling begins with repetition of simple vowels and consonants, but will gradually incorporate more complicated sounds until it becomes more like the language he hears you using. Babies love exploring all the different sounds they can make, so talk away; tell him what you are doing and point out familiar objects. Babies understand words long before they can say them, so the more you talk about the world around him, the greater his vocabulary will be when he does talk. If your baby has had a pacifier in the daytime, try to reduce its use to allow him to talk freely. By around 12 months your child may start to use simple words such as "cup" and "hot."

PENNY LAZELL
Healthcare professional

How to manage competitive mommy friends

You may find you made a new friend at prenatal classes and got on really well until you had your babies. There are moms who can't stop comparing their baby with other people's and keep pointing out things that they feel their baby does better than others. So what do you do?

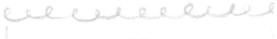

EXPERT TIP

SHE MEANS WELL

We don't always realize the effect we are having on others—as moms we want to connect, but often don't know how. Some people think giving advice or sympathy is the way to do it, not realizing that it can leave others questioning their own approach.

MIA SCOTLAND
Clinical psychologist

Becoming a mom can have a sudden and surprising effect on people. Even the woman who was a laugh and always supportive of others at the prenatal class can turn into a competitive (and often irritatingly smug) mom the minute she leaves hospital with her baby. So sometimes, you can find yourself spending too much time with a fellow mom who seems to boost her own energy and confidence by taking it from others.

These people can have uncanny knack of making you feel worse instead of better about yourself and that's not helpful during this time of significant change. Being a parent makes us extra vulnerable and, because we're bombarded with well-meaning advice everywhere we look, many women are sensitive about their mothering skills and prone to feeling insecure and unsure, because it's a time when they are building a new sense of identity. You might have been more robust about criticism before you had kids, but now you are a mother it's easy to feel undermined.

Remember she's probably not as confident as she appears to be

If you have a friend who appears to be sympathetic, while subtly chipping away at your confidence ("Still not sleeping through at 11 months? Poor you!") don't panic. This, combined with the exhaustion of being a new mom, can mean her words come across in a hurtful tone. It's very possible that she just feels secretly relieved that other moms are going through the same problems she is. But, if you feel that she thrives on your insecurity, it could be driven by her own sense of inadequacy and a need for reassurance.

First of all, talk to her. It could be that she's so obsessed with her own baby that she genuinely hasn't considered how she has been making you feel. Let her know that when she makes snippy comments about your child's progress, or lack of it, that you're hurt and it makes you anxious. If she's been doing it by accident, she'll be mortified and will probably make the effort to think before she speaks in future.

Don't be afraid to walk away

Trust your instincts however, and if they tell you it's time to move on, then do so. Enjoy the company of the moms who are encouraging, so that you can put your "friend's" influence into perspective. Instead of worrying about someone being critical, pick up the phone and call your old friends—this is a quick way of getting back your sense of self that may have been affected. Your baby will only be tiny for a few months, so share the experiences with people who support you— and remember, there are hundreds of potential new mom friends out there!

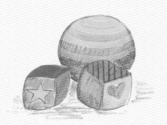

REAL LIFE

"I moved on"

"When one new friend came over for a playdate, she removed half my daughter's toys because they were 'dangerous'. Every time I saw her, it felt like she was implying I don't keep a close enough eye on my baby. I've now stopped inviting her round, and spend time with more tactful moms instead!"
SARAH, MOM TO JONAS, TEN MONTHS AND ELLA, SIX

CHAPTER THIRTEEN
FROM TEN MONTHS

Your baby's first steps will be the exciting culmination of all the skills she's learnt. While it is great to encourage her, it is also important to let her go at her own pace. The average age for first steps is around 13 months, but walking can happen as early as nine or at 18 months. Let your baby go barefoot indoors as this makes it easier for her to grip the floor. She may also be saying "mom" and "dad" now too.

ESTABLISHING GOOD EATING HABITS

It probably hasn't escaped your notice how easily a baby rice cake goes down, while a boiled carrot stick is more likely to be used for target practice. But creating good eating habits in your little one at this stage might be simpler than you think. Implement simple strategies at meal times now and you might be surprised how well your baby's eating habits continue to develop as she becomes a toddler (even if she does still throw everything she can get her hands on).

Plan meal and snacks

Offer three meals a day at set times, plus snacks and milk in between. Eating healthily goes without saying, but this will be easier if you make a weekly meal plan, as you'll know what you'll be eating in the week ahead and can shop accordingly. That way, you won't have to rely on quick fixes.

Don't insist that your baby finishes everything if she doesn't want to, as you'll just create more problems down the line—congratulate her on what she does eat. It's also important not to offer endless snacks as she may not feel hungry at mealtimes.

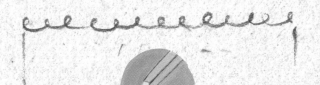

EXPERT TIP

CREATE A HAPPY EATER

Introduce new foods when you can (and remember you may need to expose your child to a new food eight to 10 times, according to the latest research, to overcome any aversion). If she rejects something, offer it again a few weeks later. Children always want what they see you eating so lead by example. Likewise, if you love your junk food, keep it to yourself—or rethink your choices. Keeping portions small sometimes helps too. Offer smaller amounts, and dish up more once she's finished. Often, toddlers don't eat all their food because there's simply too much on the plate. Around now your baby will enjoy self-feeding—which plays an important role in her mental and physical development. Encourage this as it will help with hand-eye coordination and increase her sense of independence.

CHARLOTTE STIRLING-REED
Nutritionist

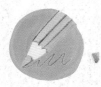

EXPERT TIP

···

POSITIVE PRAISE

If you lead by example and you're consistent in what you ask from your baby, you'll start to see results. When you do, reward that positive behavior by giving your baby lots of encouragement and approval. A powerful way to motivate your child to behave well is by giving attention in return. If you respond to her straightaway when she acts in a way you like, she'll keep behaving that way. Take the time to acknowledge what she's doing and say things like, "You're playing so nicely now." Remember, though that your child's brain is still developing and she doesn't have an older child's ability to delay gratification or see something from another child's perspective.

DR. REBECCA CHICOT

Child development and parenting expert

Keep meals fun

Young children have a short attention span, so if you want your baby to eat well, keep the focus on the food and make mealtimes fun with colorful cutlery, plates, and bibs (and keep smiling throughout, even if she's refusing everything).

THE FOUNDATION OF GOOD BEHAVIOR

Becoming a toddler is clearly not easy—not for your baby, and definitely not for you. What's even harder is working out how to go about promoting good behavior while getting a handle on the more challenging stuff, and without crushing her emerging independence either.

In fact from the moment you start getting routine into your baby's life, you begin to create boundaries. These routines show your baby that you're in charge and you're meeting her needs—and that in turn builds a trust between you. Then, as your child moves towards toddlerhood, you can start putting positive barriers in place.

Experts agree that teaching your child to set limits on her behavior is one of the most valuable things you can do for her. As well as helping her to develop self-control, it's also the foundation she needs to go on to build fulfilling relationships with other people. So say things like, "Play nicely" or "Touch gently."

Even though your baby doesn't know the difference between right and wrong, start putting techniques in place that will work in the years to come. If she does something that is potentially dangerous, such as pulling on a tablecloth, gently say "no" and redirect her to a safer activity. Baby proofing your home will make it a lot easier for you to allow your little one some freedom of movement so she can explore her world a little (see page 93).

TRIPS TO THE PLAYGROUND

It's important that your baby gets plenty of fresh air, even when you don't feel like going out, because vitamin D is a crucial bone-building, immune-boosting vitamin that the body creates through exposure to the sun. Even in winter, your child gets a little bit of sun whenever she is outside in daylight—20 minutes is enough. Fresh air also clears out her lungs, and going outside usually leads to some exercise, which will boost everyone's mood. Your child is less exposed to other people's bugs outside, so make your way to your nearest park. The fresh air will also help her sleep better. Research suggests that being outside in the late afternoon could help babies and children to rest better at night, because it sets their circadian rhythm, or internal body clock.

Layering in the cold

If it's cold, wrap up warm because being cold stresses a child's immune system, which makes her more susceptible to illness. Layer her up with long-sleeved T-shirts, hats, and cardigans, rather than putting her in one big coat that can cause her to overheat. Remove layers as necessary. Take off wet hats and socks as soon as possible, too, as they cause body temperature to drop quickly.

Clean up when you are home

If you've been out with your crawling baby and she has come back dirty, make sure you wash her hands and clean any dirty toys. Hand washing can reduce your baby's chances of getting ill, especially once she's mobile and picking up more germs.

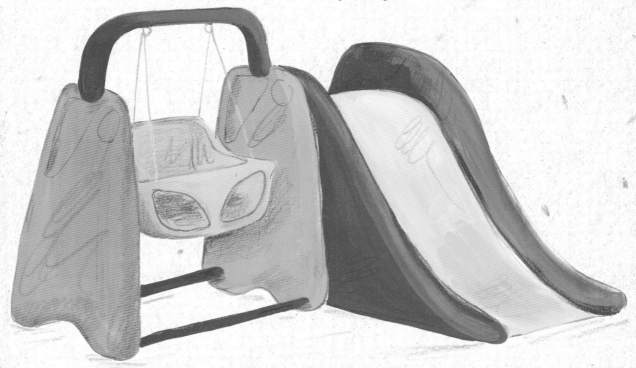

How can I get a good night's sleep?

You know the drill—baby wakes, you wake—but what about when she's dropped off again and you can't? A recent survey found the average mom loses nearly 44 days' sleep in the first year of her baby's life, and yes, broken nights can be a shock to the system, but there are ways to maximize the amount of rest you get and become a smarter sleeper.

Anxiety is a big cause of tossing and turning, often because new moms feel worried about their responsibilities. However it's a vicious circle: the more tired you are, the more anxious you become, and the worse you sleep. Pare down your to-do list to the bare essentials and use any baby-free time to unwind. Read a magazine, have a soak in the bath, take a nap: in short, do anything that clears your mind and slows your breathing.

Take comfort in the fact that you're resting, even if you're not sleeping. And it might be the last thing you feel like doing, but exercise, such as a daily walk or, if you have the time, a swim, can relieve stress and regulate your body clock. This in turn means you'll have better quality sleep.

Eat regularly and don't stay up too late
We've all been there. Relishing a few hours of grown-up time, but that second wave of energy you experience once your baby goes to bed is down to increased adrenaline because your body is overtired. To avoid this, get into good habits: eat breakfast within 30 minutes of waking, for example, as it stabilizes blood-sugar levels and regulates the production of the sleep-inducing hormones serotonin and melatonin. It's also wise not to eat dinner too late. It's tempting to wait until your baby is in bed, but if you can, eat around 7pm, and try to be in bed by 9pm at least a few nights a week.

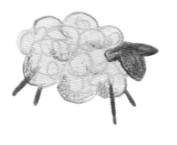
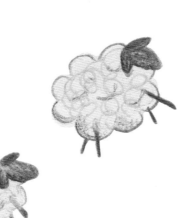
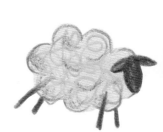

If you just can't drop off

Switch off your TV/laptop/cell at least an hour before you sleep—artificial light can lower levels of melatonin (and raise levels of the stress hormone that wakes you up, cortisol). Try playing white noise to soothe both of you—not just your baby. You can buy special machines that replicate the sound of rain falling or wind through trees, but an electric fan is just as good.

If you wake too early

Morning light seeping into your room can make you more alert, so install a blackout blind or wear a sleep mask. If you still can't sleep, try not to stress. If you only have an hour before you need to get up, you probably wouldn't slip back into a deep sleep anyway. Instead relax and try some breathing exercises. Breathe deeply through your nose, then exhale through your mouth for a count of ten. Repeat to achieve a state of deep relaxation. Once you take the pressure off yourself, you may find you drop off naturally anyway.

If your baby has a sudden sleep regression

When your baby is ill, you might get a night so bad you are exhausted. Once your baby starts to sleep through, your own body reconditions itself to need more sleep. So, when you have a bad night, it can feel worse than in the first few weeks. The only thing you can do is clear your diary and conserve energy during the day. Extreme lack of sleep can impair mental capacity to such an extent that it's hard to function, so avoid driving. If you can get someone to sit for a couple of hours while

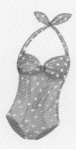

REAL LIFE

"My regular swims have helped"

"When Rosa was ten months old, I rediscovered swimming—it really helped me relax and gave me some time to myself too. I started going to the gym for a quick swim in the late afternoons while my partner looked after Rosa, and it really helped my quality of sleep. I don't think I'll ever stop, and I've toned up too!"
SYLVIA, MOM TO ROSA, TWO

you nap, then do. If not, rest as much as you can by relaxing when you can on the sofa, and going for a nap when your baby is asleep in her crib.

YOUR BABY'S GROWING
AWARENESS AND
THE FEARS IT CAN BRING

·······································

INCREASING BUMPS AND SCRAPES
AS YOUR BABY
STARTS TO EXPLORE

CHAPTER FOURTEEN:
FROM ELEVEN MONTHS

Your baby's walking skills will continue to develop over the next months as he works towards walking on his own, though some babies will just be standing and crawling at this point. You can also start teaching your baby about shapes with toys that require him to put different shapes through matching holes.

UNDERSTANDING YOUR BABY'S FEARS

As children grow and discover the world around them, they not only develop their skills and personalities, but their fears too. Anxiety about certain situations and scenarios is perfectly normal and it usually changes according to your baby's stage of development. Most fears are protective instincts inbuilt to the human psyche when the brain registers that a situation could be unsafe. Common anxieties in younger children up to the age of 18 months include fear of strangers, loud noises, and being left on their own. This is a developing process, so when a baby learns to crawl and begins to move away from

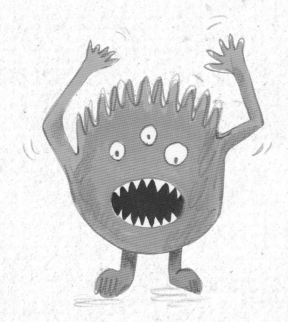

his mother, separation anxiety is likely to kick in to promote proximity and safety. Of course, it is very early days now but in the future, as a toddler grows up, his imagination develops, so he may become anxious of the dark and imaginary creatures might permeate his nightmares, from monsters under the bed to ghosts. Fears manifest themselves when a child is coping with being in a room on his own, away from his mom. His brain registers that he feels unsafe. These fears are linked with the evolution of the imagination too. A toddler has no real concept of what is real and what is imaginary; children only begin to learn the difference from around eight years of age.

Toddlers are biologically programmed to be anxious about food, especially new flavors and textures. Children rely on mom to know what food is safe to eat and what food is not—this is a natural instinct. Interestingly, actions speak louder than words—especially facial expressions. So if you say "eat your yummy banana" but pull a disgusted face, your toddler is hard-wired to be cautious of the banana. Similarly, if you tell him not to be scared of something, but you look afraid, your child will pick up on this.

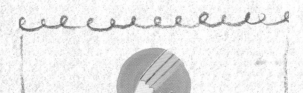

EXPERT TIP

· ·

COMBATING FEAR

Think about how you react to your child's anxiety. Children need to feel secure and safe and their fears are very real to them. Rather than making light of worries, explore them and help them feel reassured.

DR REBECCA CHICOT

Child development and parenting expert

DEALING WITH BUMPS AND SCRAPES

By this stage your baby will be moving around exploring. It will be amazing to see him develop, but all this movement is tough on his skin too. He'll be making his way over all types of terrain—carpets, grass, and wooden floors—potentially rubbing, burning or cutting his hands or knees especially. It's a good idea to protect your child's skin (you can buy products that resemble legwarmers, to help protect his knees). And if he does get a minor cut or graze, clean it thoroughly, and protect it with a plaster or dressing. Most cuts and grazes are minor and can be easily treated at home. If you are concerned that a wound may be becoming infected, for example if there is pus or the surrounding skin looks very red and inflamed then see your doctor.

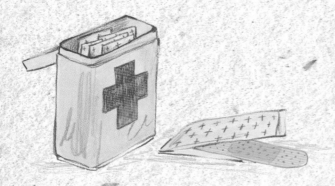

EXPERT TIP

HOW TO TREAT A GRAZE

For minor scrapes, just wash the area with lots of warm water. If the wound is bleeding, place a sterile gauze pad or clean cloth over it and press with your fingers to stop the bleeding first.

Dab around it with an antiseptic, dab it dry and cover it with a sterile dressing. You can also get spray-on or brush-on dressings to keep out germs out; ask your local pharmacist to recommend one.

If you're worried at all about your baby's injury call your doctor, but if the cut keeps bleeding or there's a gap between the edges of the wound or if there is a possibility of a foreign body (such as a piece of glass), go to an urgent care facility or your local hospital emergency department. If your child's immunizations aren't up to date, tell your doctor or the hospital.

DR PHILIPPA KAYE
Family doctor

QUICK FIX

BE PREPARED

Keep a well-stocked first aid box in a cupboard at home (see page 114) and another small one in the car in case of emergency.

How to get your sexy back

If sex has been at the bottom of your must-do list for a while, try targeting some of the more common emotional barriers. The key issues can be frustration, resentment, exhaustion, anxiety, and that sense of being "all loved out" from pouring all your affection on your baby.

Frustration is common

If you've spent all day caring for your baby, only for your partner to fall asleep in front of the TV, it's normal to feel that it's your life that's taken the biggest hit. Meanwhile, he's probably dealing with the pressure of providing for his new family and may be working extra hard, rather than helping with the baby. The apparent imbalance of power can cause resentment while you are on maternity leave. Another area of resentment can build if you aim to split the domestic chores equally, but feel that you do more. Discuss how you both feel about your set-up.

Secondly, because women's libidos are more closely connected with our physical state, tiredness is more likely to put women off sex than men. If your partner gets more sleep than you, explain that there needs to be a balance. Let him know that if you get more rest, you'll feel like you're being cared for and desired.

If you're home with your baby all day, it's normal to find that you have enough hugs from your baby during the day. By the time your partner gets home, you're craving time on your own. Explain that it's not because you don't fancy him, it's just that you need to have 20 minutes by yourself.

Feeling anxious about sex

Coming to terms with your new identity and body can make you feel anxious too. Having morphed into a baby-nurturing machine, it's hard to get back into a sexier mindset. But remember that sex is about how you feel, not just how you look. To nurture your sexy side, keep a diary of when you're thinking about any kind of intimacy and try to spot the triggers.

Make time together

Once you've talked through your emotions, make time together for sex, even if it's just while you settle into life as parents and have a different relationship routine. Book a sitter for an evening or ask someone to look after your child for a few hours, so that you both have the house to yourself; the sooner something gets on the calendar, the sooner you can start getting excited and in the mood for some time together.

Stay flexible and don't set strict goals and you don't have to have full intercourse. There's no need to give yourself targets such as having an orgasm either. In fact, having no expectations makes things more relaxed, which leaves you more sexually responsive. Try to steal little moments and simpler pleasures, such as showering together, cuddling on the sofa or having a lunch date. Finally, realize that, as with any phase in your life, this is temporary. If you're having less sex, it's a trade-off for everything else amazing that's happening right now.

CHAPTER FIFTEEN
AT TWELVE MONTHS

Get your camera ready—as well as celebrating your baby's first birthday it could be around now that she takes her first steps. Some babies start earlier, some later, but between nine and 18 months, most babies gain their balance and learn to walk. Your child should have her one-year scheduled well visit (or check up) with her pediatrician, covering language and learning, safety, diet, and behavior.

REACHING KEY MILESTONES

When she's learning to take her first steps hold both her hands to help her practise walking while keeping her balance; encourage her to keep her heels flat. Don't worry if walking by herself doesn't happen right away, she'll get there in her own time. Once she's got her walking/waddling skills sorted, you will need to take her to buy that first pair of shoes to protect her feet properly when you're out and about. It's important to watch her closely while she's walking around and never let her go up or down stairs on her own.

First real words too
Her constantly developing language skills mean she'll probably be babbling a lot too. She's been taking in everything you've been saying during her first year, she may say her first word around her first birthday. Even if she doesn't, you'll start to see a lot of development as her speech develops at her own pace over the next year or so—she will understand much more than she can say, for example identifying people, body parts, and objects, and will also be able to point out familiar things.

Over the coming year and beyond, rather than getting your child to copy you parrot fashion, which she may find hard work, prompt her to say the word. Instead of saying "say ball, say ball," point to her ball and say "this is a ..." and pause. She'll delight in telling you the answer. Don't pressurize her or worry if she isn't word perfect. There'll be plenty of mispronunciations; at this stage she needs all the encouragement you can give her. So, for example, if she points to a cat and says "tat," praise her by saying "That's right, a cat," and reinforce the correct pronunciation without her realizing what you are doing.

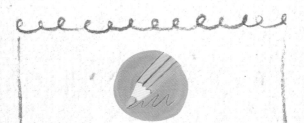

EXPERT TIP

NEW SKILLS MEAN NEW GAMES

Just after her first birthday your baby will become interested in ball play, thanks to her fast-developing motor skills and hand-eye coordination. First, she'll roll and then she'll throw before moving onto kicking. Your child loves crayons and painting at this age too, because it's fascinating for her to make marks on paper (cause and effect). It also helps improve the pincer grip, which will eventually help her write. So, hand over that crayon and let her loose on some paper...

PENNY LAZELL
Healthcare professional

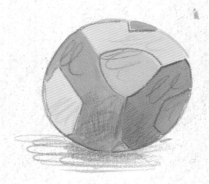

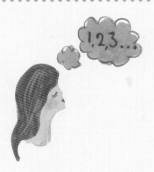

REAL LIFE

"My stay-calm trick"

"When Rowan used to have tantrums as a toddler, they seemed to last forever—and I would become upset and flustered, especially if we were out somewhere. I felt people were judging me and I didn't know how to handle him. But I started saying to myself, 'Remember, you're the adult and you're in control', and it really helped me stay calm and rational. As a result Rowan would calm down too. It sounds silly, but it helped me!"
STELLA, MOM TO ROWAN, 4

TODDLER TANTRUMS MAY BEGIN

There's no escaping a tantrum, and sometimes, little people and meltdowns go hand in hand. So next time your toddler goes into full-blown tantrum mode, remember, it's all totally normal, and every mom has been there at some time. Remember your child is expressing how she feels in the only way she can because she doesn't yet have the skills to hold back or express herself in any other way. Anger and frustration collide, and the result can be fairly dramatic.

Whatever the reason for your child's outburst, remind yourself that she's acting on impulse. So while sometimes you can anticipate a trigger and

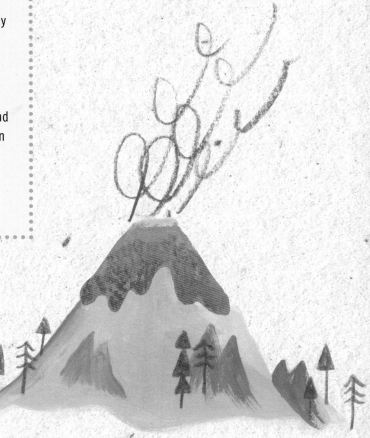

avoid a tantrum before it starts (for example, keep her well-fed, well-rested, and hydrated) at other times there's not a lot you can do. Even in the most unlikely situations, you may be able to detect tiredness, boredom, frustration, or hunger as the root cause. At other times your child may just be unsettled by a change in routine or is reacting to stress around her. But tantrums often reach such an intensity so quickly because of your child's inability to see life from anyone else's perspective. What looks like a small, screaming banshee is just a tiny person who feels something is wrong, but doesn't know how to put it right, so wants you to do it for her.

MANAGING TANTRUMS

If your toddler has a meltdown, she's simply communicating that she wants her needs met and she can't understand why you're not doing anything about it. When she has an outburst in a public place, it's easy to feel as if other people are judging you, but the truth is that they're probably not. Of course if you're in a restaurant or somewhere where there are other people with a reasonable expectation of peace, you can gently try to remove her from the situation and look after her elsewhere. If your little one is tired, hungry, or unwell, these things will affect her behavior, so try to deal with these issues swiftly, calmly, and rationally, even if you're feeling flustered.

Having trouble staying calm?
Try breathing in for a count of five and out for a count of ten—it's the ultimate calmer and de-stresser. The last thing you want to do is to reach similar levels of frustration and anger as your toddler, because she'll pick up on it. You're the adult and need to stay calm, and this will (fingers crossed), help to calm her.

EXPERT TIP

GO EASY ON YOURSELF
Putting too much pressure on yourself can lead to more than just stress: it can contribute to the onset of depression. So, if you are feeling the pressure, talk to someone you trust, whether that's a friend, relative, or professional, about how you're feeling. The more we can have conversations about what real life is really like, the more we can reduce the expectations we put on ourselves. As mothers we don't have to be perfect, we just have to be good enough. If you're doing your best and your baby is happy, you're doing great.

MIA SCOTLAND
Clinical psychologist

····· There's no such thing as the perfect mom ·····

Yes, we all know the "rules"—from not letting babies have too much screen time, to not giving them convenience food—and yet we all break them. No-one is the perfect parent, because there's no such thing. Like every other mom, we're all working hard and sometimes we just can't tick all the boxes. Although our children are, for the most part, happy and healthy, it's difficult to ignore the nagging guilt that we should be doing it all better.

The pressure to do everything right is everywhere; in newspaper articles, social media posts, baby groups, TV adverts, and most of all in ourselves. In a recent *Mother&Baby* survey, 77 per cent of moms said they felt the pressure to be perfect, and 75 per cent said this pressure had increased since becoming a parent. Furthermore, over half of you admitted to having parenting-related meltdowns as you strive for perfection.

Be a good enough parent

It's time to shift the focus from striving to be "perfect" to striving to be "good enough." Perfection doesn't exist. It is just a way in which we put a huge amount of unnecessary pressure on ourselves. Women are having children later in life and so the build-up to parenthood is greater, plus the rise of social media offers an easy life-comparison tool—and we rarely come out better by comparing ourselves to other people. So ensure your baby is happy and healthy, have fun with your amazing toddler, and enjoy the next 18 years (and many more).

REAL LIFE

"Look at all the positives!"

"When I had my first baby, I was obsessed with reading up on how to look after him and would panic if I thought I didn't make the best purée, or pick the best nappy. I was forever secretly comparing his development with other babies and telling myself I wasn't doing enough to teach him new things. But after a year I realized I was being way too hard on myself. I wasn't doing anything wrong and in fact, I was a brilliant mom. Berating myself about the small stuff was only distracting me from just enjoying my fantastic, happy, healthy baby. I'm still a bit of a perfectionist, but I look at all the positives now, rather than worrying about what my 'failings' might be."

ELLA, MOM TO GEORGE, THREE AND ALEX, 11 MONTHS

NOTES

WHAT AN EXCITING YEAR! HERE'S LOOKING FOWARD TO THE NEXT ONE...

8 TO 12 MONTHS

MONTH 8

MONTH 9

His skill set is constantly growing, try to encourage him to try new toys and ones that help him to develop his constantly evolving problem-solving skills.

MONTH 8

Your baby will be developing a pincer grip and will become more interested in grabbing things and picking them up.

His mouth muscles are still developing as he masters chewing and learning to swallow, this can mean he gags a bit, but just stay nearby to reassure him.

MONTH 9

MONTH 10

MONTH 9

MONTH 10

Your baby's first steps can be as early as nine or at 18 months.

MONTH 8

Separation anxiety can set in at any time from six to 18 months, but often starts around now as your baby starts to recognize you as a separate person.

Your baby may start cruising between bits of furniture—encourage this by placing a few chairs in a line for him to move from one to the other.

Try exposing him to new foods and remember that he might have to try new things up to ten times to overcome an aversion to new flavors and textures.

You can see your baby's personality evolving and with this he could also be building up fears and anxieties, which you'll need to do your best to reassure him about.

MONTH 11

MONTH
11

His increased movement will mean bumps and scrapes are increasingly common. Keep any wounds clean and protected.

MONTH 12

This can be the start of toddler tantrums. Try to anticipate what triggers them to avoid them in the first place, but remember he's just trying to communicate his needs in the only way he knows how.

MONTH
12

Many babies' first words will be spoken around their first birthday.

MONTH 12

He'll be increasingly interested in new games that hone his growing hand-eye coordination, including ball games and drawing with crayons.

NOTES

USE THESE PAGES TO MAKE NOTES ON YOUR
AND YOUR BABY'S JOURNEY AND PLAN THE
EXCITING TIMES AHEAD.

NOTES

GLOSSARY

allergen A substance that causes an allergic reaction.

amniotic fluid The fluid surrounding a foetus within a woman's amniotic sac where an unborn baby grows and develops.

automated auditory brainstem response (AABR) screening test One of two hearing tests that will be offered to all newborns before leaving the hospital. Sounds are played to the baby's ears. Doctors measure how the hearing nerve responds and can identify babies who have a hearing loss.

baby immunization program A schedule of treatments, usually injections, designed to protect children against a number of diseases.

baby-led feeding Rather than giving babies purées when it is time to feed them solids, baby-led feeding is when parents let babies feed themselves with soft foods.

baby-proofing The safety assessment and securing of potentially dangerous hazards around your home or back yard for babies who are beginning to crawl or walk.

bacterial infection Illnesses that occur when harmful forms of bacteria multiply inside the body. Ranging from mild to deadly, most can be prevented by good sanitation or cured by antibiotics.

botulism Botulism is a rare but serious illness caused by a bacterium which occurs in soil. It produces a toxin that affects your nerves. Food-borne botulism comes from eating foods contaminated with the toxin.

cardiopulmonary resuscitation/CPR An emergency procedure of chest compressions and rescue breaths used on people who are not breathing properly or if their heart has stopped.

cognitive behavioral therapy/CBT A form of talking therapy which is used to treat anxiety or depression by changing the way you think and behave.

circadian rhythm The daily cycle of biological activity observed in humans and many living organisms.

colostrum The thin yellowish fluid, rich in antibodies, that is secreted from the nipples just after giving birth.

contact dermatitis This occurs when your skin reacts to a particular substance—either an irritant or an allergen—like detergents, cosmetics or metals.

cortisol Known as "the stress hormone" because stress activates cortisol secretion in the body.

cradle cap Common and harmless condition, similar to dandruff, found in babies under 12 months old. While predominantly a condition of the scalp, it can be found on the face, neck or even the back of the knees (see also *seborrhoeic eczema*).

cruising After babies learn to stand, their first steps are usually accompanied by them moving around a room—or "cruising"—by clinging on to items of furniture for support.

engorgement The painful overfilling of the breasts with milk, usually the result of an imbalance between supply and baby demand.

eczema Dry, red, itchy or cracked skin that can itch or bleed. Extremely common.

estrogen A group of hormones secreted by the ovaries. Responsible for regulating a woman's reproductive cycle, including suppressing the menstrual cycle of a breastfeeding mother.

expressing The squeezing of milk out of the breasts, usually by means of an electric pump, so it can be stored and fed it to an infant at a later time.

fontanelle The areas of an infant's head where the soft membrane has yet to harden into a fully formed skull.

flat-head syndrome Name given to the condition when a part of a baby's head becomes flattened due to continued pressure on one spot.

frenulum The tight piece of skin between the underside of the tongue and the floor of the mouth. In cases of tongue-tie, this could sometimes prevent a baby from breastfeeding effectively.

iron Iron is an essential mineral, with several important roles in the body. For example, it helps to make red blood cells, which carry oxygen around the body.

IUD/intrauterine device One of two contraceptive devices that makes it difficult for a fertilized egg to implant in your womb. One type is a small plastic and copper contraceptive device that is inserted in the uterus and the other releases a hormone that's a type of progesterone.

Both are inserted vaginally by a doctor. The hormone-containing IUD makes it difficult for a fertilized egg to implant in your womb. It also thickens the mucus in your cervix making it difficult for sperm to enter your womb.

latched on When a breastfeeding baby's mouth sucessfully engages with the nipple and areola and begins to suck and draw out milk.

let-down reflex The name given to the process when the milk draws down and into the nipple when a baby is breastfeeding.

mastitis Often-painful inflammation of the breast. Can become infected which means that bacteria grow in the inflamed tissues.

meconium The dark browny-green first poo that a newborn baby passes, made up of various fluids ingested inside its mother's womb.

melatonin A natural hormone given as a supplement to help you sleep. However, this may be harmful to your baby if you are pregnant or breastfeeding. Seek medical advice.

Moro reflex The name given to the reflex action of the arms and legs by a young infant (up to four months of age) when startled by a sudden loud noise. It is named for the person who first described it—Ernst Moro.

motherese Baby talk used by a mother to communicate with her infant.

otoacoustic emission (OAE) screening test One of two hearing tests that will be offered to all newborns before leaving the hospital. A probe is placed in the ear and sounds are played. If a baby hears normally, an echo is reflected back into the ear canal and is measured by the probe.

oxytocin Female hormone released in large amounts during labor—aiding contractions—and after stimulation of the nipples. It is seen as the facilitator for both childbirth and breastfeeding.

pediatrician Doctor who specializes in the treatment of babies and children.

pincer grip The name for the "grasping" movement, whereby a small object can be held by an infant.

PP-PTSD/postpartum post traumatic stress disorder The name given to a set of reactions to a traumatic experience during childbirth.

PPD/postpartum depression A common form of depression brought on by childbirth.

progesterone Hormone produced in the ovaries, placenta and adrenal glands of a woman that helps prepare her for conception and pregnancy and regulates the monthly menstrual cycle.

prostagladin receptors Prostagladins regulate the female reproductive system and are involved in the control of ovulation, menstrual cycle, and induction of labor.

reflex action Involuntary actions that babies make that in time (usually around three months later) will be replaced by conscious movements.

reflux The term given to the process when the milk your baby has swallowed comes back up into his food pipe. See also *spit-up*.

salmonella Bacteria that causes gastrointestinal problems, usually affecting the small intestine. A common reason for diarrhea in young children.

sebaceous glands Glands in the facial skin which produce a waxy or oily matter called sebum (see below); these can become enlarged, blocked or infected in children, causing a rash.

sebum Oily substance secreted by the sebaceous glands that helps prevent hair and skin from drying out.

separation anxiety Very common reaction by young infants, usually screaming or crying, to when parents—especially mothers—or close carers leave them unattended for any length of time.

serotonin A neurotransmitter that is involved in the transmission of nerve impulses around the brain, seen as the key to mood regulation.

seborrhoic eczema See *cradle cap*.

SIDS/sudden infant death syndrome Also known as crib death, a diagnosis made when an apparently healthy baby dies without warning and for no clear reason.

spit-up A small amount of milk that a baby brings up after a feed. Often occurs in conjunction with wind.

sterilize To make something free from bacteria.

swaddle Practice of wrapping babies safely and in a specific way in a cloth or blanket with the aim of calming them. The head should never be covered—seek help to learn how to swaddle safely and correctly.

thrush A vaginal yeast infection. Can also be an oral infection—a fungal infection of the mouth.

tongue-tie Piece of tissue between the underside of the tongue and floor of the mouth. Can restrict the movement of the tongue in breastfeeding, but can be alleviated with a simple procedure.

transition to solid foods The traditional approach of feeding babies purées before slowly introducing different food types.

tryptophan An amino acid found in milk (and some other foods) that can raise serotonin levels and is thus said to aid sleep.

tummy time In order to develop the strong neck muscles that a baby needs in order to learn to sit, crawl, and walk, they need time on their front when awake—"tummy time."

umbilical stump After a baby is born the umbilical cord is clamped and cut leaving an umbilical stump that eventually dries up and drops off.

virus/viral infection A virus is a small infectious agent that replicates only inside the living cells of other organisms. Diseases caused by viruses include flu and colds.

vernix The white substance that covers and protects the skin of the fetus and is still all over a baby's skin at birth.

vitamin D A vitamin essential for the absorption of calcium and the prevention of rickets in children.

white noise A sound that contains every frequency within the range of human hearing in equal amounts, "white noise"—a sound similar to radio or TV static—is believed to replicate the sounds heard in the womb and keep a baby quiet.

wrap sling A piece of woven or stretchy jersey-type fabric that you wrap and tie around your body so your baby is held securely. There have been warnings about the possible dangers of the carriers and suffocation risks.

MEET THE EXPERTS

Lara Palamoudian is an editor who specializes in health and wellbeing, parenting and women's lifestyles. She is a former Deputy Editor of *Mother&Baby* and was also Editor of its sister title *Pregnancy&Birth*.

Dr Rebecca Chicot is co-founder of *The Essential Parent Company*. She has a doctorate in child development and parenting and is a member of the Association of Infant Mental Health. Rebecca worked for many years at BBC Television in London making science documentaries for BBC1. www.essentialparent.com

Dr Philippa Kaye currently works as a general practitioner in North London. She has an interest in women's, children's, and sexual health. She is also an author and contributor to books about women and children. www.drphilippakaye.com

Denyse Kirkby is a registered midwife (RM), registered midwifery teacher (RMT), Higher Education Academy (HEA) fellow, and United Kingdom Public Health Register (UKPHR) registered public health practitioner (PHP) and author. www.djkirkby.co.uk

Penny Lazell has worked in the NHS since 1984. She is a Registered General Nurse (RGN) and Health Visitor (RHV) A quialified medical worker who lends support and offers advice to parents. She is also a qualified Midwife and Neonatal Nurse and also runs private health visits and a children's sleep consultancy. www.healthvisitor4u.com

Mia Scotland is a Clinical Psychologist, specialising in pregnancy, birth, and parenthood. She is the author of *Why Perinatal Depression Matters* and runs a trauma and depression clinic in Melton, as well as hypnobirthing classes. She travels around the country running workshops for midwives and doulas on the psychology of pregnancy and birth. www.yourbirthright.co.uk

Tina Southwood had a long career as a nanny to newborns, and there's nothing this sleep consultant and night nanny doesn't know about getting your baby to sleep. www.sleep-baby-sleep.co.uk

Charlotte Stirling-Reed is a registered nutritionist who has experience working with the NHS, the media, and with private organisations. Charlotte runs a nutrition consultancy firm called *SR Nutrition* and specializes in pediatric nutrition and nutrition during pregnancy. www.srnutrition.co.uk

Mother&Baby is the UK's No. 1 Pregnancy, Baby, and Toddler Magazine—and the home of all the latest expert advice covering every aspect of becoming a mom. *Mother&Baby* is sold in the UK, Ireland, Australia, China, Croatia, Indonesia, Poland, Serbia, Singapore, Turkey, India, and beyond. Find out more about *Mother&Baby* at www.motherandbaby.co.uk

FURTHER RESOURCES

American Academy of Pediatrics
National organization that represents 64,000 pediatricians nationwide. The website gives age-appropriate advice for children.
www.healthychildren.org

Choose My Plate.gov: Pregnancy & Breastfeeding US Department of Agriculture website that provides dietary guidelines for women who are pregnant or breastfeeding.
www.choosemyplate.gov/moms-pregnancy-breastfeeding

Hand to Hold
Nonprofit organization that provides advice for parents of preemies or other babies who need to stay in the neonatal intensive care unit (NICU).
www.handtohold.org

La Leche League
Providing information and support for breastfeeding mothers.
www.llli.org

Multiples of America
National network of more than 300 local clubs spread across the US for parents of twins, triplets, quadruplets and other multiples.
www.nomotc.org

National Alliance for Breastfeeding Advocacy
Nonprofit organization that is the primary lobbying group in support of breastfeeding in the US, The group encourages all women to breastfeed their babies.
www.naba-breastfeeding.org

National Alliance on Mental Illness
Nonprofit organization that helps people find support regarding mental health issues.
www.nami.org

National Partnership for Women & Families
Nonprofit organization that supports fairness in the workplace for men and women. They lobby for reproductive health rights, for expansion of FMLA, and for paid leave for mothers and fathers. nationalpartnership.org

Parents Without Partners
Nonprofit organization devoted to single parents and their children.
www.parentswithoutpartners.org

Postpartum Support International
Nonprofit organization dedicated to helping women who suffer from depression during and after pregnancy by increasing public awareness and by educating healthcare professionals.
www.postpartum.net

Safe to Sleep
Public education campaign with information about ways to reduce the incidence of SIDS.
www.nichd.nih.gov/sts/

US. Consumer Product Safety Commission
Government agency working to ensure that products sold in the US don't cause injury or death.
www.cpsc.gov

US Lactation Consultant Association
Association for international board-certified lactation consultants (IBCLCs).
www.uslca.org

INDEX

An Hachette UK Company
www.hachette.co.uk

First published in Great Britain in 2016 by
Hamlyn, a division of
Octopus Publishing Group Ltd
Carmelite House
50 Victoria Embankment
London EC4Y 0DZ
www.octopusbooks.co.uk

Distributed in the US by
Hachette Book Group
1290 Avenue of the Americas
4th and 5th Floors
New York, NY 10020

Distributed in Canada by
Canadian Manda Group
664 Annette St.
Toronto, Ontario, Canada M6S 2C8

ISBN 978 0 60063 378 5

Printed and bound in China

10 9 8 7 6 5 4 3 2 1

Publishing Director Stephanie Jackson
Editor Pauline Bache
Copy-editor Jemima Dunne
US consultant Lisa Fields
Designer Isabel de Cordova and Jaz Bahra
Illustrator Abigail Read
Senior Production Manager Pete Hunt

Octopus Publishing Group would like to thank
Claire Irvin, Busola Evans, Lara Palamoudian,
Sally Saunders, Dr Rebecca Chicot, Dr Philippa
Kaye, Denyse Kirkby, Penny Lazell, Mia Scotland,
Tina Southwood, and Charlotte Stirling-Reed.